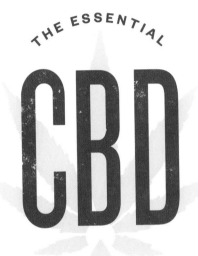

THE ESSENTIAL

CBD

COOKBOOK

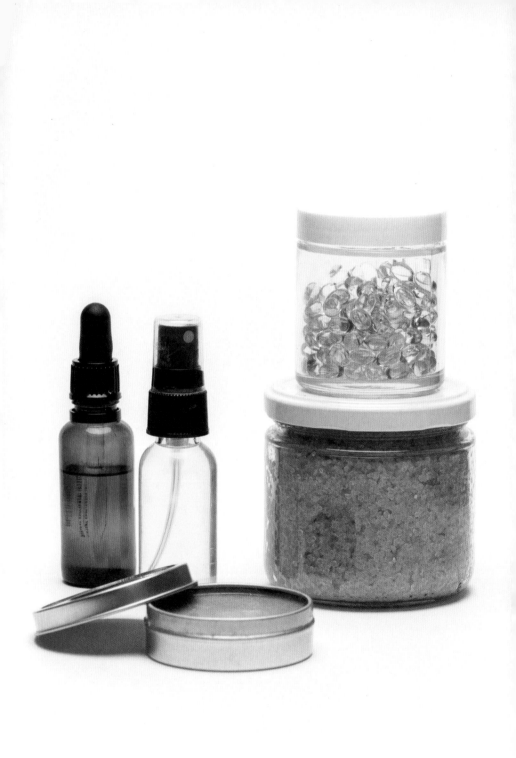

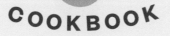

THE ESSENTIAL CBD COOKBOOK

HARMONY BOOKS
NEW YORK

CONTENTS

INTRODUCTION

We all want to feel our best. For some, that means eating well, exercising, and taking vitamins. Others rely on natural remedies like medicinal roots or herbs. CBD is another useful tool to keep your mind and body healthy.

What is CBD?

Cannabis has been used in medicine for thousands of years in Asia to treat ailments such as rheumatism, gout, and malaria. It wasn't until the early nineteenth century that researchers began studying its benefits and medicinal applications. It is believed that the cannabis used during this time was low in THC and high in CBD and therefore excluded the psychoactive effects. Over time, more studies were conducted, and in the 1980s, CBD was shown to be effective in treating epileptic seizures. In the 1990s, researchers discovered the endocannabinoid system, a complex biological system that allows cannabis to interact with the receptors in our bodies.

Even though both CBD and THC are derived from the cannabis plant, they are very different in what they do. Cannabidiol (CBD for short) is a molecular component of the cannabis plant, a cannabinoid. THC is also a cannabinoid, but unlike THC, CBD does not contain any form of the psychoactive component that gives you that "high." CBD is non-psychoactive and nonaddictive. There are CBD products that contain some THC, and for some people, THC aids the body's receptors to accept CBD.

We now know that there are numerous benefits to using CBD both topically and internally. CBD has antifungal and antibacterial properties, with research showing that it is effective at killing bacteria and even superbugs. In patients with epilepsy or multiple sclerosis, seizures and spastic pain dissipate with the usage of CBD. CBD works as an anti-inflammatory, which aids those with chronic pain issues.

There are several studies that show how CBD acts on receptors in our nervous system, and how our bodies perceive pain, inflammation, and anxiety differently when using CBD. It can also offer relief from diseases such as autoimmune diseases, Parkinson's, diabetes, and psoriasis, among others. For people looking for an all-natural alternative to pharmaceuticals, this supplement could be the solution.

How do you use CBD?

Multiple success stories and accounts serve as evidence of its usefulness in treating anxiety, depression, pain, and insomnia. In some cases, CBD can even increase energy levels. Even if your ailments are not severe, you can use CBD to treat symptoms to your own comfort level. CBD oil is now readily available, and ingesting it orally is becoming more popular. It can be taken in many ways, such as capsules, vapor, patches, lotions, sprays, oils, and tinctures. Some people ingest the oil and tinctures on their own, but they can be added to a variety of foods to help mask the earthy, bitter taste that some people find unpleasant. In the following recipes you will find a variety of healthy "edibles" you can make. CBD can also be used topically. It can provide localized relief and can help relieve skin conditions such as acne or eczema. Use the oil by itself, make it into a lotion, infuse it with Epsom salts for a bath, or add it to a body scrub to give yourself a spa treatment with a little stress management and pain relief rolled into one.

Because CBD is such a new and burgeoning industry, more scientific research is needed in order to pinpoint a universal dosage. Like every other natural remedy out there, it may take a little while for your body to become attuned to its effects, and it doesn't work in the same way for everyone. But it's worth experimenting a little with dosing—a dropper full of oil or a slather of lotion might be what works for you.

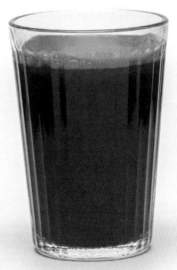

BUYING CBD

When it comes to buying CBD, be sure to do your research or buy it from a legitimate source. There are many "CBD" products that falsely claim to include CBD. There are sites online where you can check the validity of some of these CBD companies and their claims.

Full-Spectrum CBD

Full-Spectrum CBD contains everything from the plant, including all the terpenes, flavonoids, and cannabinoids, and because nothing is removed, all those components work together to become highly effective. This is known as the "entourage effect." Full-Spectrum CBD is more beneficial than CBD isolate.

vs.

Broad-Spectrum CBD

Broad-Spectrum CBD lies somewhere in the middle of CBD isolate and full-spectrum CBD. It contains all the components of full-spectrum CBD but with THC removed, so that it contains the "entourage effect" benefits of full-spectrum CBD.

vs.

CBD isolate

Isolate CBD is the purest form of CBD. It removes all other compounds found in the cannabis plant including terpenes, flavonoids, and other cannabinoids. It is the only CBD that is extracted from hemp and is tasteless and odorless. This is a good oil to use for making topicals.

THC in your CBD?

You may have come across some CBD products with THC in them. Depending on what you want from your supplement, you could get one with THC or THCa.

THCa is another cannabinoid in the cannabis plant and isn't psychoactive. It is the raw acid form of THC and works the same way that THC does to aid CBD in interacting with our body's receptors. The only catch is, if you let this oil/tincture heat up in your car or in your house on a hot day, or even in cooking, it activates the psychoactive component, so it is best to keep this in the fridge and/or add it to your food after cooking, just before serving.

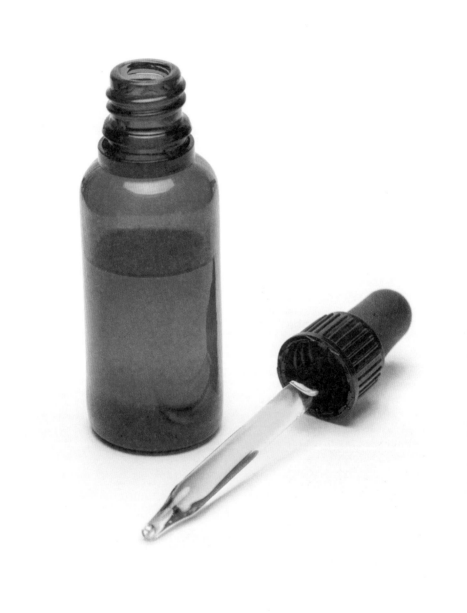

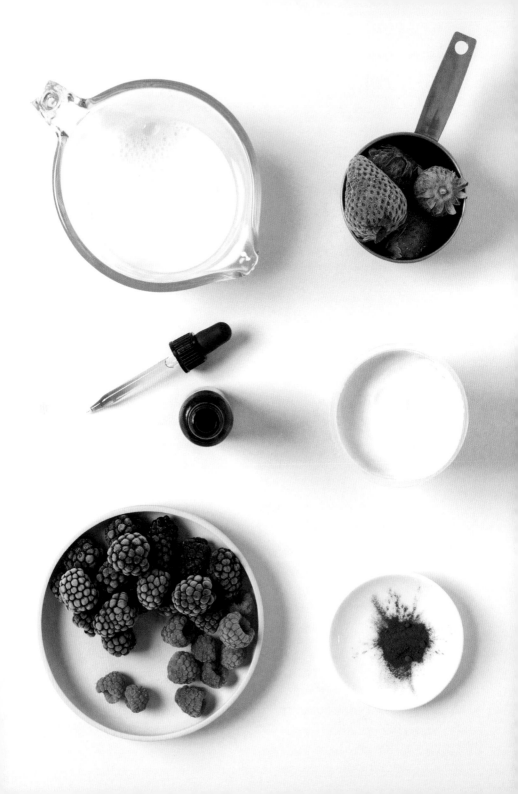

HOW TO USE/DOSAGES TIPS

Tips on cooking with CBD

- Start with small doses. Make sure the taste is at the level you want before adding more.
- CBD is best ingested with other beneficial fats, such as ghee or coconut milk. Your body absorbs it more easily with these fats.
- CBD can be added to almost everything you eat, but be careful when using heat with it. At temperatures higher than 160°C/325°F, you can lose the beneficial qualities of terpenes, the essential oils present in CBD. Heating CBD oil also tends to bring out its bitterness. You should be careful with CBD that contains any sort of THC, as the heat may activate it.
- If using CBD in smoothies or juices, be sure to blend and stir it in thoroughly before and while you are drinking. CBD oils or tinctures are mainly oil-based, and in water-based juices and smoothies the oil will separate from the water.

Tips on dosage

Most CBD oils have dosages on their products, usually 1 dropperful, but what works for one person may be different for another. The dosage should be based on the concentration of CBD, the weight of the person, the person's sensitivity to the product, and the condition that's being treated.

- A good rule of thumb to follow is to take 1 to 6 mg of CBD for every 10 pounds of body weight, and based on the severity of the person's condition.
- Start small, about 5 to 10 mg per serving, 2 to 3 times a day. Take a little more if you don't feel any effect.
- Consult your doctor! As with any drug or supplement, consult your doctor or health practitioner.
- When making topical products, typically about 300 to 500 mg of CBD oil is used per 1 ounce of topical product.

All the recipes in this book are based on CBD oil with 1000 mg concentration of CBD and an average weight of 150 to 240 pounds. Please adjust accordingly.

JUICES & SMOOTHIES

Juices and smoothies are one of the quickest and easiest ways to add CBD to your diet.

Mint Lacto-Fermented Soda • Beet & Orange Juice
Lacto-Fermented Lime Soda • Mint, Apple & Pear Juice
Watermelon Mint Agua Fresca • Lacto-Fermented Berry
Soda • Hibiscus Vanilla Agua Fresca • Cucumber &
Watermelon Juice • Coconut Turmeric Smoothie
Green Smoothie Bowl • Ginger Greens Smoothie
Strawberry Chia Smoothie • Peach Blueberry Blue Magic
Mixed Berry Smoothie Bowl • Strawberry Oat Smoothie
Greener than Grass Smoothie • Ginger & Peach
Smoothie • Mango & Cacao Smoothie Bowl
Blueberry Chia Smoothie • Acai Smoothie Bowl
Blueberry Smoothie Bowl

MINT LACTO-FERMENTED SODA

Makes: 1 quart (2 cups whey) - Preparation: 30 minutes - Fermentation: 2 to 3 days

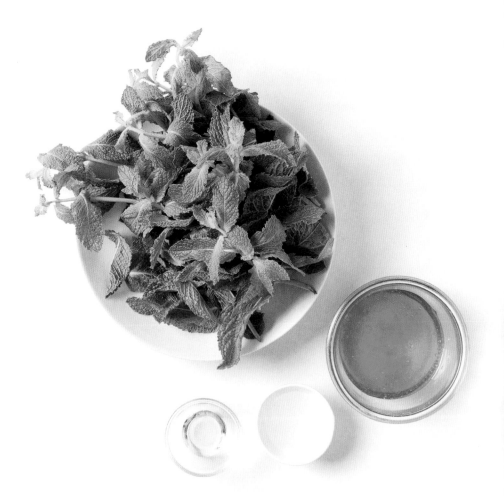

YOU NEED
2 tablespoons whey • 2 bunches of mint (about 1½ ounces) • ¼ cup honey
100 mg CBD oil (about 4 dropperfuls)
For the whey: 10½ ounces natural whole yogurt or milk kefir

Makes for a great refreshing, healthful soda

D *Aids digestion* **H** *Hydrating* **M** *Mineral rich*

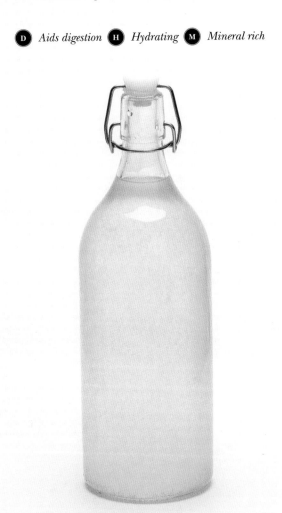

For the whey, line a strainer with 4 layers of muslin and set over a large bowl. Add the yogurt, cover, and leave for 4 to 6 hours or chill overnight. Liquid whey will drain into the bowl. For the soda, bring the mint, honey, and 1½ cups water to a boil, then simmer for 20 minutes. Cool, then strain the mixture over a bowl. Pour the strained mint mixture, CBD oil, and whey into a 1 liter flip-top bottle. Top with filtered water and close. Leave for 2 to 3 days until you see fizziness at the top. Chill. Serve cold.

BEET & ORANGE JUICE

Makes: 1 cup - Preparation: 5 minutes

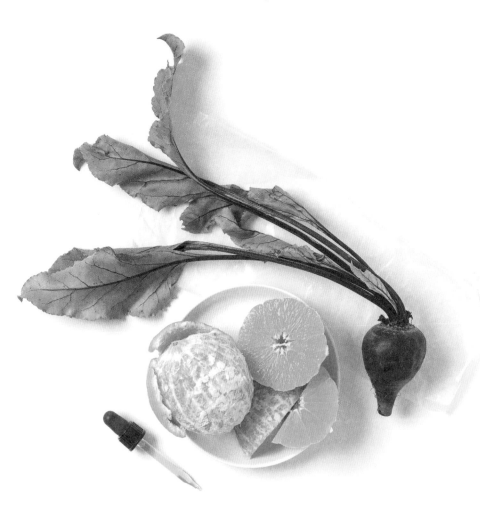

YOU NEED

¼ large beetroot, peeled

2 navel oranges, peeled, seeded, and quartered

22 mg CBD oil (1 dropperful)

Beetroot juice is loaded with nitrates and promotes healthy blood flow.

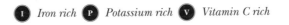 **I** *Iron rich* **P** *Potassium rich* **V** *Vitamin C rich*

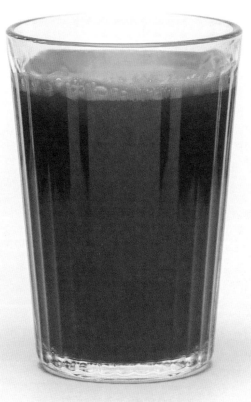

Place the beetroot and oranges in a juicer and juice, then add the CBD oil and stir
together well. Add ice, if you like.

LACTO-FERMENTED LIME SODA

Makes: 1 quart - Preparation: 20 minutes - Fermentation: 2 to 3 days

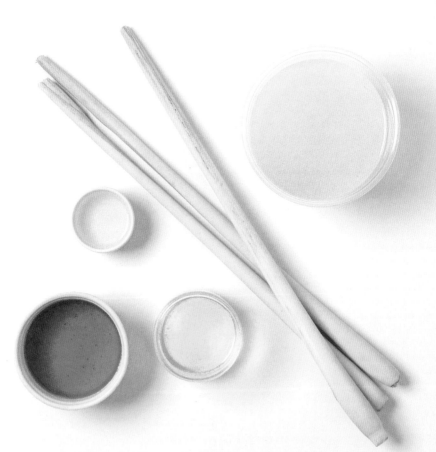

YOU NEED

3 lemongrass stalks, tender parts chopped • ½ cup honey

1½ cups lime juice • 100 mg CBD oil (about 4 dropperfuls)

2 tablespoons whey (see page 14)

The vitamin C in both the lemongrass and the lime helps to relieve any respiratory problems.

 Infection fighting **B** *Anti-bloating* **I** *Immunity boosting*

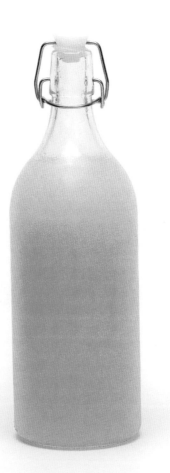

Bring 1½ cups water, the lemongrass, and the honey to a boil in a pan. Reduce the heat and simmer for 20 minutes, stirring occasionally. Leave to cool to room temperature. Strain the mixture through a fine-mesh strainer over a large bowl. Pour the syrup, lime juice, CBD oil, and whey into a 1-quart flip-top bottle. Top with filtered water and close. Leave to ferment for 2 to 3 days until you see fizziness at the top. Chill and serve cold. Drink a glass a day until you know your dosage limits.

MINT, APPLE & PEAR JUICE

Makes: 1 cup - Preparation: 5 minutes

YOU NEED

10 mint sprigs, leaves picked • 1 Granny Smith apple, cored and quartered

1 Honeycrisp apple, cored and quartered

2 pears, Bosc or d'Anjou, cored and quartered

22 mg CBD oil (1 dropperful)

This is a great juice to help aid digestion.

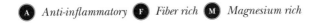 **A** *Anti-inflammatory* **F** *Fiber rich* **M** *Magnesium rich*

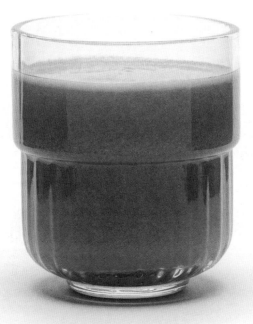

Place all the ingredients, except for the CBD oil, in a juicer and juice. Add the CBD oil and stir thoroughly. Serve immediately.

WATERMELON MINT AGUA FRESCA

Makes: 2 cups without ice - Preparation: 30 to 40 minutes

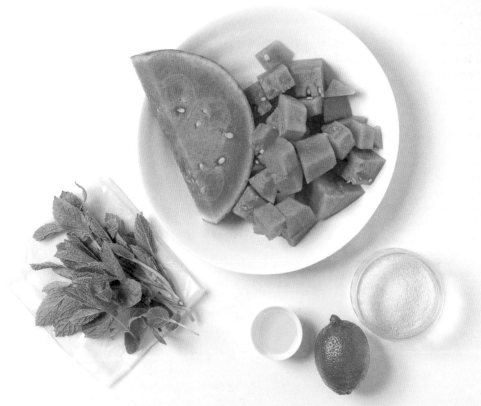

YOU NEED

2 tablespoons granulated sugar, or more, depending on your taste

½ ounce mint • 1⅓ pounds watermelon, peeled and chopped

juice of 1 lime • 100 mg CBD oil (about 4 dropperfuls)

This drink is very hydrating.

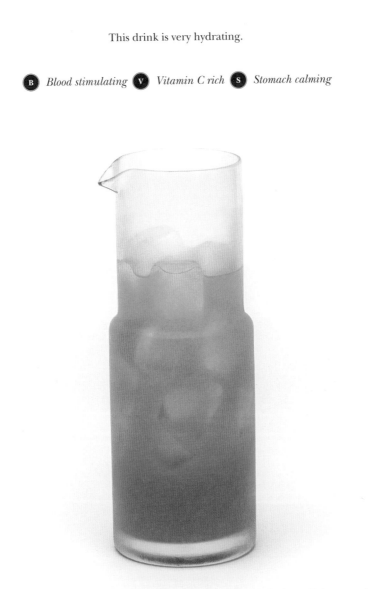

Combine the sugar, mint, and 2 tablespoons hot water and stir until the sugar is dissolved. Leave for 30 minutes or longer to infuse. Blend the watermelon in a blender along with the lime juice. Strain through a strainer into a pitcher, then stir in the mint syrup and CBD oil. Store in a jar or pitcher for 3 to 4 days in the fridge. Serve chilled or over ice.

LACTO-FERMENTED BERRY SODA

Makes: 1 quart - Preparation: 20 minutes - Fermentation: 2 to 3 days

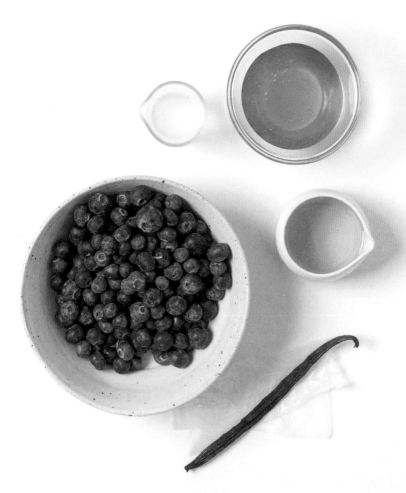

YOU NEED

½ pound blueberries • 1 vanilla pod, split in half lengthwise

½ cup honey • 2 tablespoons whey (see page 14)

100 mg CBD oil (about 4 dropperfuls)

Blueberries are one of the fruits highest in antioxidants.

 Immunity boosting **B** *Blood pressure lowering* **A** *Anxiety relieving*

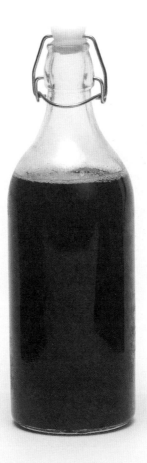

Bring 3 cups of water and all of the ingredients, except for the whey and CBD oil, to a boil. Reduce the heat and simmer for 20 minutes, stirring occasionally. Leave to cool to room temperature. Strain the mixture through a fine-mesh strainer over a large bowl. Then pour the mixure, the CBD oil, and the whey into a 1-quart flip-top bottle. Top with filtered water, leaving about 1½-inch space and close. Leave to ferment for 2 to 3 days until you see fizziness at the top. Chill and serve cold.

HIBISCUS VANILLA AGUA FRESCA

Makes: 1 quart - Preparation: 15 to 20 minutes

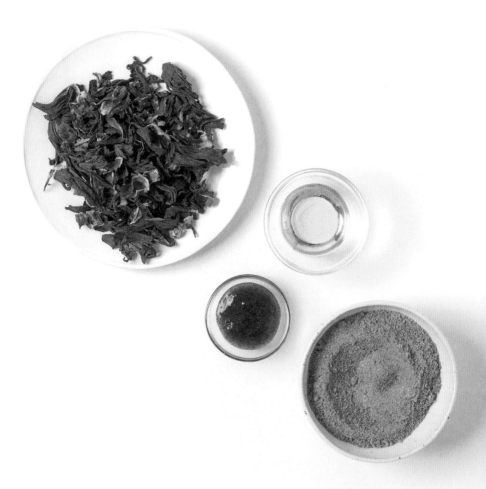

YOU NEED

1 ounce dried hibiscus flowers • 1½ ounces coconut sugar

2 teaspoons vanilla bean paste • 100 mg CBD oil (about 4 dropperfuls)

Hibiscus boosts liver health.

C *Cholesterol lowering*   **A** *Antibacterial*   **W** *Weight loss promoting*

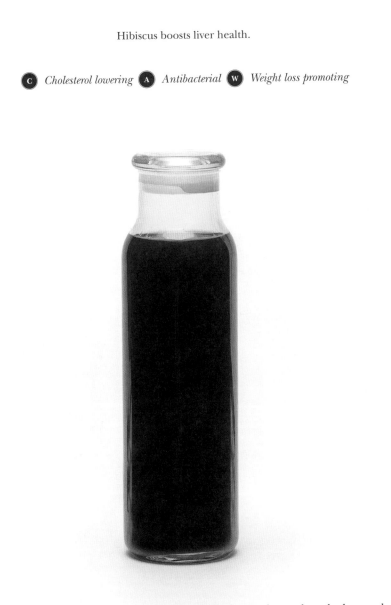

Bring the hibiscus and 1½ cups water to a boil in a pan, then reduce the heat and simmer for 15 minutes. Add the coconut sugar and vanilla and stir until dissolved. Leave to cool, then add the CBD oil together with 1 cup water. Store in a jar or pitcher for 3 to 4 days in the fridge. Serve chilled or over ice.

CUCUMBER & WATERMELON JUICE

Serves: 1 - Preparation: 5 minutes

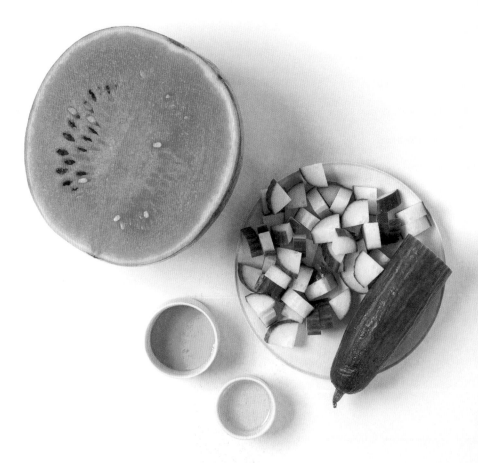

YOU NEED

5 ounces watermelon, peeled and cubed

1 cucumber, roughly chopped

1 teaspoon honey (optional) • 100 mg CBD oil (about 4 dropperfuls)

This drink can help aid in weight loss.

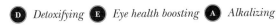

D *Detoxifying* **E** *Eye health boosting* **A** *Alkalizing*

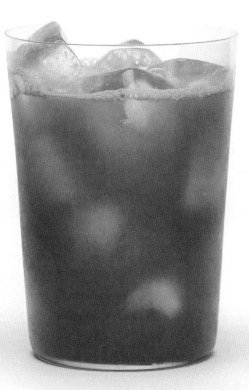

Place the watermelon and cucumber in a juicer and juice. Stir in the honey (if using) and CBD oil until combined. Serve chilled or over ice.

COCONUT TURMERIC SMOOTHIE

Serves: 1 - Preparation: 5 minutes

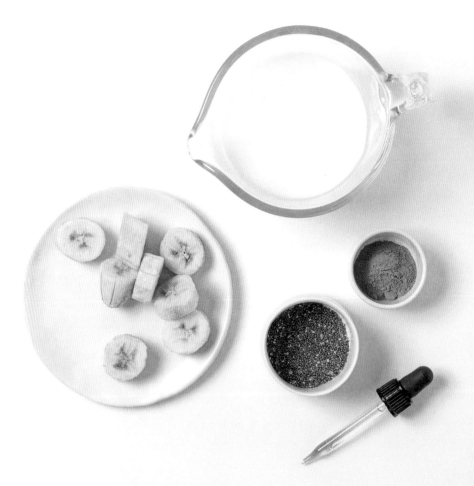

YOU NEED

1 cup canned coconut milk, plus extra as needed • ½ frozen banana

1 teaspoon ground turmeric • 1 teaspoon chia seeds

22 mg CBD oil (1 dropperful)

Chia seeds are a great source of omega-3 fatty acids.

 Brain boosting **C** *Cholesterol lowering* **P** *Potassium rich*

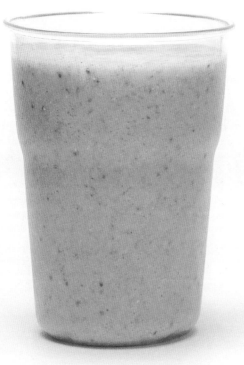

Combine all the ingredients in a blender and blend until smooth. Add more coconut milk as needed to get the blender moving. Serve immediately.

GREEN SMOOTHIE BOWL

Serves: 1 - Preparation: 5 minutes

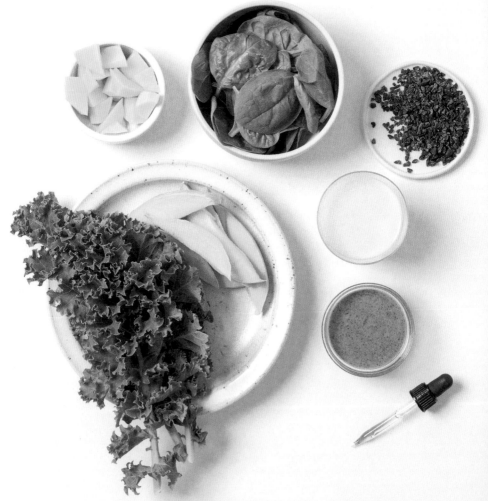

YOU NEED

3¼ ounces frozen mangoes, chopped, plus 1½ ounces fresh mango chunks

1 ounce baby spinach • 3 kale leaves, de-stemmed

½ cup unsweetened almond milk • 2 tablespoons almond butter

22 mg CBD oil (1 dropperful) • 1 tablespoon cacao nibs

This is a great way to make a smoothie into a meal.

 Nutrient dense **I** *Iron rich* **H** *Heart health boosting*

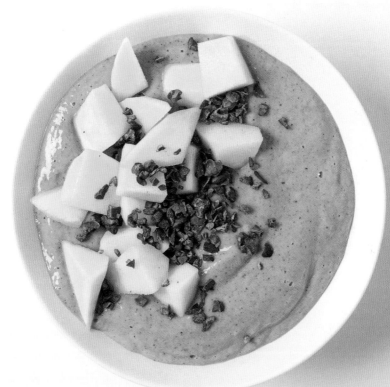

Combine the frozen mangoes, spinach, kale, almond milk, almond butter, and CBD oil in a blender and blend until thick but smooth. Pour into a bowl and top with the cacao nibs and the fresh mango chunks. Serve immediately.

GINGER GREENS SMOOTHIE

Serves: 1 - Preparation: 5 minutes

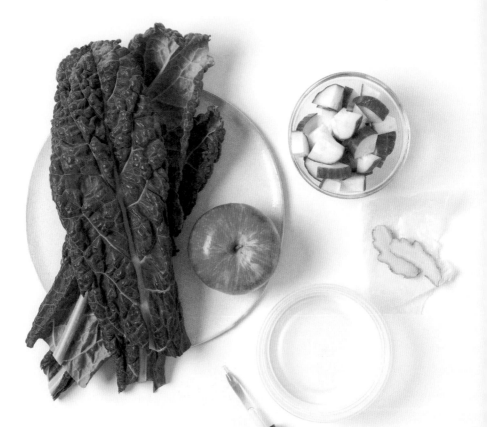

YOU NEED

4 lacinato kale leaves, de-stemmed

4½ ounces chopped cucumber • 1 small Gala apple, peeled and chopped

½–1½-inch piece of fresh ginger, peeled and roughly chopped

½ cup filtered water, plus extra as needed

22 mg CBD oil (1 dropperful)

Ginger can help reduce muscle soreness.

 Gingivitis preventing *Energizing* *Cholesterol lowering*

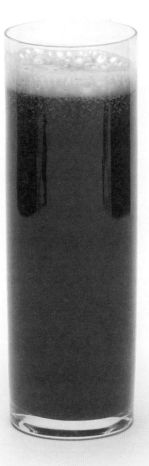

Combine all the ingredients in a blender and blend until smooth. Use more water as necessary. Serve immediately.

STRAWBERRY CHIA SMOOTHIE

Serves: 1 - Preparation: 5 minutes

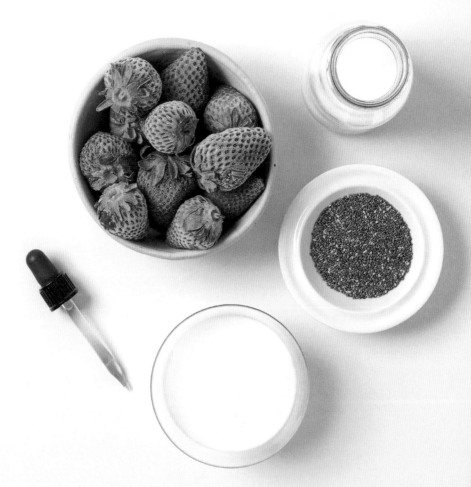

YOU NEED

9 ounces frozen strawberries • ½ cup natural yogurt

5½ ounces milk • 2 tablespoons chia seeds

22 mg CBD oil (1 dropperful)

Strawberries are high in vitamin C.

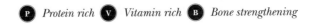

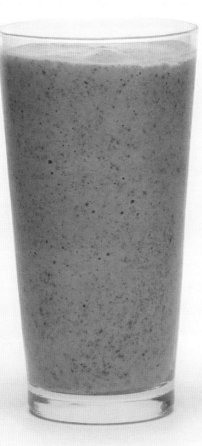

Combine all the ingredients in a blender and blend until smooth.
Serve immediately.

PEACH BLUEBERRY BLUE MAGIC

Serves: 1 - Preparation: 5 minutes

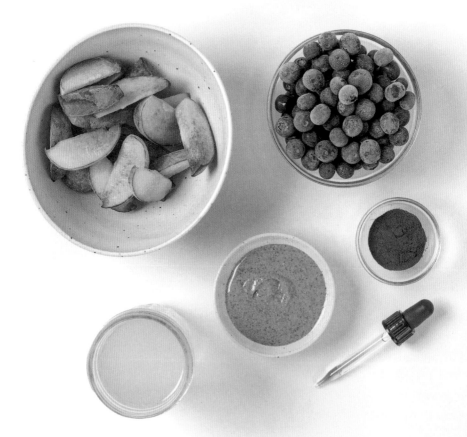

YOU NEED

5¼ ounces frozen peaches • 5¼ ounces frozen blueberries

2 teaspoons spirulina • 6 ounces coconut water

2 tablespoons almond butter • 22 mg CBD oil (1 dropperful)

This is a great source of vitamin E.

 Bone strengthening *Metabolism boosting* *Detoxifying*

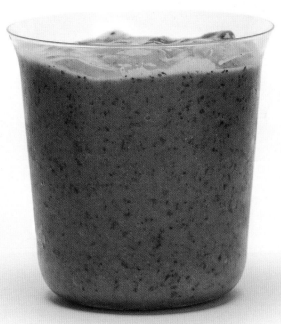

Combine all the ingredients in a blender and blend until smooth.
Serve immediately.

MIXED BERRY SMOOTHIE BOWL

Serves: 1 - Preparation: 5 minutes

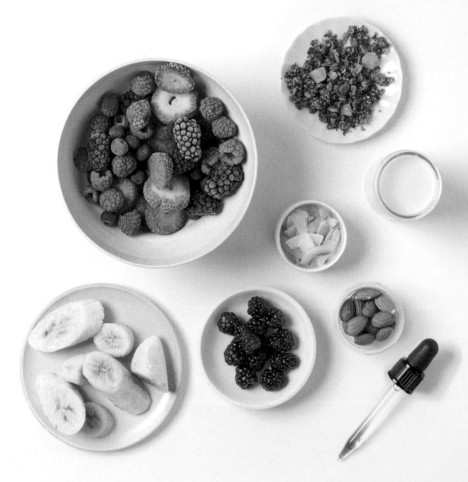

YOU NEED

7 ounces frozen mixed berries • 1 frozen banana • 6 ounces unsweetened almond milk • 22 mg CBD oil (1 dropperful) • toppings of your choice, such as toasted almonds, toasted coconut, granola • 1½ ounces blackberries

This bowl is high in potassium.

 Cholesterol lowering **I** *Inflammation fighting* **N** *Nutrient rich*

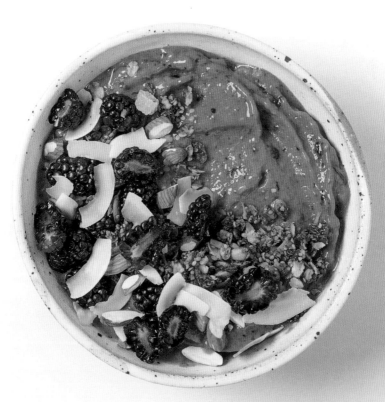

Combine the mixed berries, banana, almond milk, and CBD oil in a blender and blend until thick but smooth. Pour into a bowl and top with your choice of toppings and the blackberries. Serve immediately.

STRAWBERRY OAT SMOOTHIE

Serves: 1 - Preparation: 5 minutes

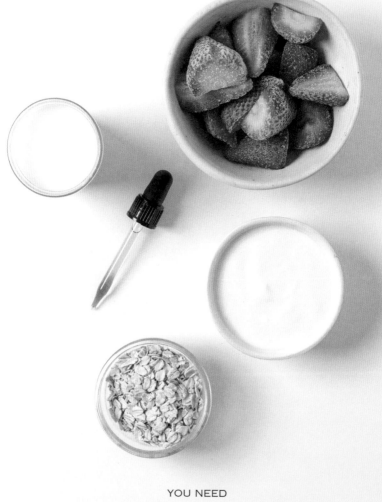

YOU NEED
4¼ ounces frozen strawberries • 1 ounce rolled oats
6 ounces vanilla yogurt • 6 ounces milk
22 mg CBD oil (1 dropperful)

The oats will help keep you satiated.

C *Calcium rich* **P** *Probiotic* **B** *Blood pressure lowering*

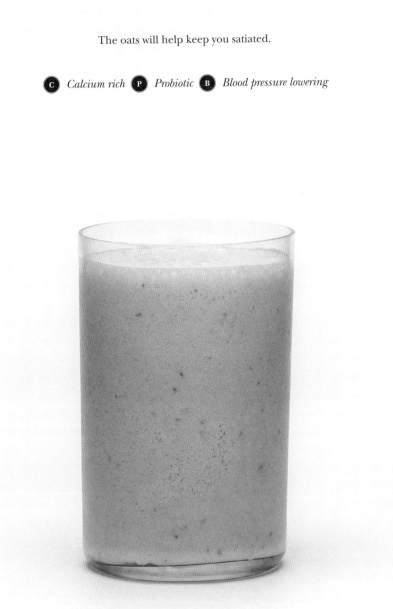

Combine all the ingredients in a blender and blend until smooth.
Serve immediately.

GREENER THAN GRASS SMOOTHIE

Serves: 1 - Preparation: 5 minutes

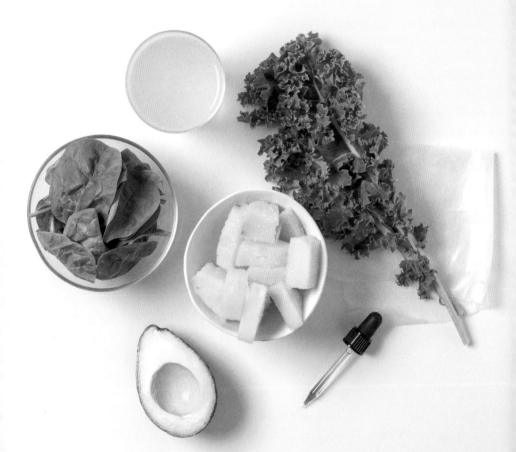

YOU NEED

1 ounce baby spinach • 2 kale leaves, roughly chopped

7 ounces frozen pineapple chunks

½ avocado, peeled, pitted, and roughly chopped

1 cup coconut water • 22 mg CBD oil (1 dropperful)

The dark leafy greens in this smoothie may prevent heart disease.

 Vitamin C rich *Vitamin K rich* **E** *Eye health boosting*

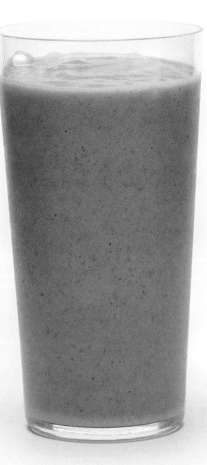

Combine all the ingredients in a blender and blend until smooth.
Serve immediately.

GINGER & PEACH SMOOTHIE

Serves: 1 - Preparation: 5 minutes

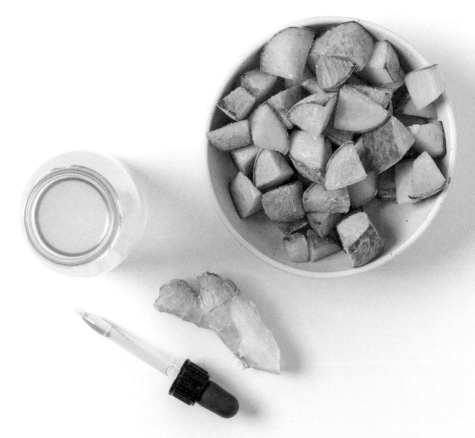

YOU NEED

5 ounces frozen peach cubes • 1 cup coconut water

½–1¼-inch piece of fresh ginger, peeled and roughly chopped

22 mg CBD oil (1 dropperful)

The peaches in this drink may help your skin maintain moisture and protect it from sun damage.

 Allergy relieving **D** *Detoxifying* **P** *Potassium rich*

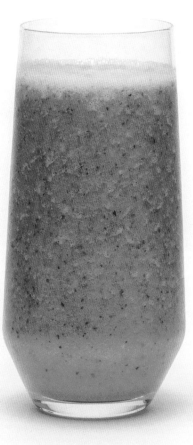

Combine all the ingredients in a blender and blend until smooth.
Serve immediately.

MANGO & CACAO SMOOTHIE BOWL

Serves: 1 - Preparation: 5 minutes

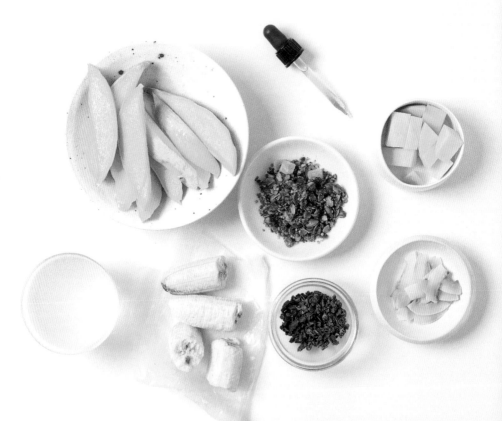

YOU NEED

6½ ounces frozen mango chunks, plus 1½ ounces fresh mango chunks

1 frozen banana, roughly chopped • ½ cup coconut water

22 mg CBD oil (1 dropperful) • 1 tablespoon cacao nibs

toppings of your choice, such as toasted coconut, granola

Coconut water is a natural source of electrolytes.

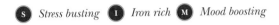 **S** *Stress busting* **I** *Iron rich* **M** *Mood boosting*

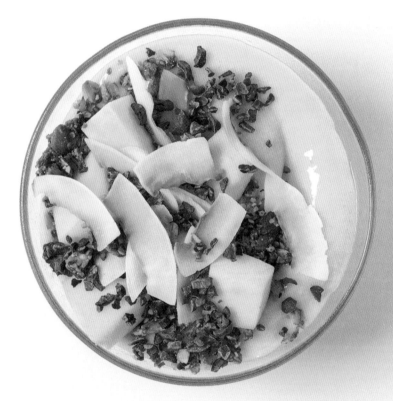

Combine all the ingredients, except for the fresh mangoes, cacao nibs, and toppings, in a blender and blend until smooth. Top with the fresh mangoes, cacao nibs, and toppings of your choice. Serve immediately.

BLUEBERRY CHIA SMOOTHIE

Serves: 1 - Preparation: 5 minutes

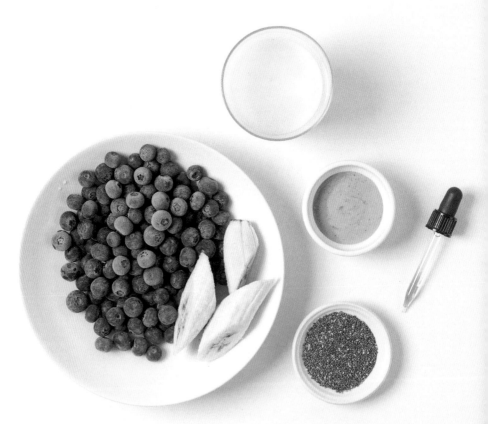

YOU NEED
6½ ounces frozen blueberries • ½ frozen banana, roughly chopped

6 ounces milk or alternative milk • 1 tablespoon smooth peanut butter

1 tablespoon chia seeds • 22 mg CBD oil (1 dropperful)

Blueberries are known to be an antiaging food.

 Cholesterol lowering **B** *Brain boosting* **P** *Protein rich*

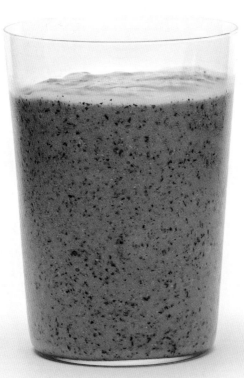

Combine all the ingredients in a blender and blend until smooth.
Serve immediately.

ACAI SMOOTHIE BOWL

Serves: 1 - Preparation: 5 minutes

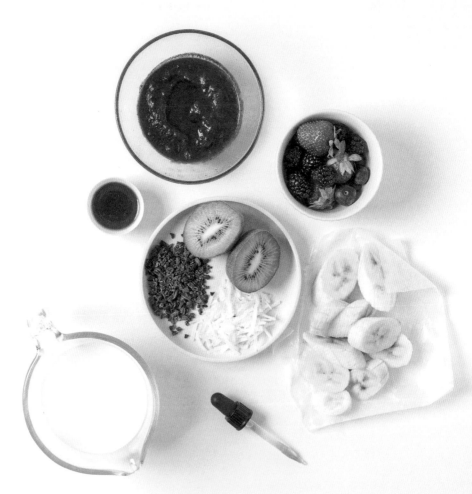

YOU NEED

7 ounces frozen, unsweetened acai puree

1 frozen banana, roughly chopped • 1 cup milk or alternative milk

1 tablespoon maple syrup • 22 mg CBD oil (1 dropperful)

toppings of your choice, such as shredded coconut, kiwifruit, berries, cacao nibs

Acai contains a lot of heavy fats, which is great for CBD intake.

 Memory boosting **D** *Aids digestion* **A** *Antioxidant rich*

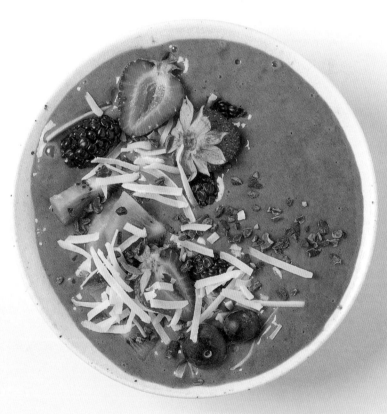

Combine all the ingredients, except for the toppings, in a blender and blend until thick but smooth. Top with the toppings of your choice. Serve immediately.

BLUEBERRY SMOOTHIE BOWL

Serves: 1 - Preparation: 5 minutes

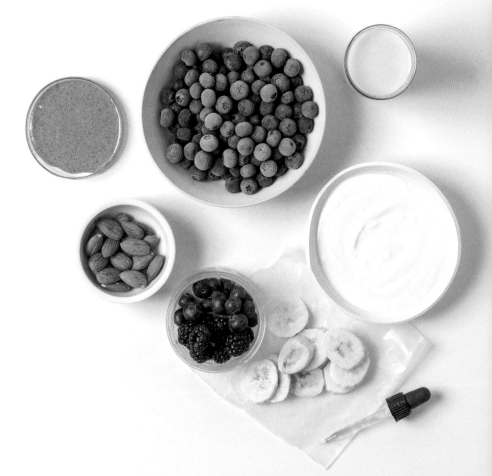

YOU NEED

7 ounces frozen blueberries • ½ cup almond yogurt

½ cup unsweetened almond milk • 1 tablespoon almond butter

22 mg CBD oil (1 dropperful)

toppings of your choice, such as fresh berries, toasted almonds, banana

Yogurt is a great vegetarian source of omega-3 fatty acids.

 Vitamin E rich **C** *Calcium rich* **B** *Bone strengthening*

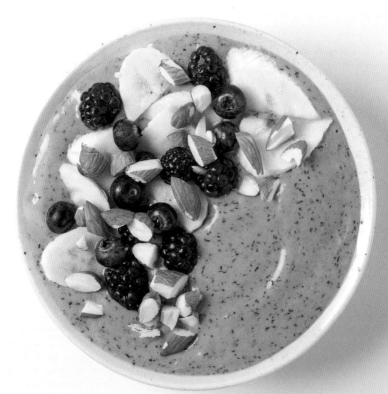

Combine all the ingredients, except for the toppings, in a blender and blend until thick but smooth. Top with the ingredients of your choice. Serve immediately.

TEAS & TONICS

The following recipes are soothing and healing teas and tonics, which are great for reducing anxiety.

Orange Cardamom Tisane • Vanilla Matcha Latte

Iced Matcha with Mint • Iced Citrus Toasted Barley Tea

Lemon Verbena & Lavender Tisane • Licorice Root

Chocolate Tisane • Goji, Cinnamon & Anise Tisane

Fennel Seed & Apple Tisane • Iced Vanilla Chai Latte

Iced Matcha Lemonade • Immunity Booster

Digestive Tonic • Cleansing Tonic • Inflammation Fighter

Hydrating Tonic • Calming Tonic

ORANGE CARDAMOM TISANE

Serves: 4 - Preparation: 5 minutes - Steeping: 10 minutes

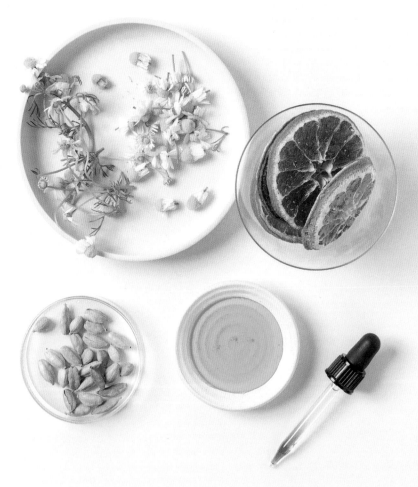

YOU NEED

4 dried orange slices • 1 tablespoon cardamom pods, crushed

1 tablespoon dried chamomile flowers

1 tablespoon orange blossom honey • 60 mg CBD oil (3 dropperfuls)

This calming tea can help lower stress levels.

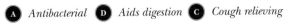

(A) *Antibacterial* (D) *Aids digestion* (C) *Cough relieving*

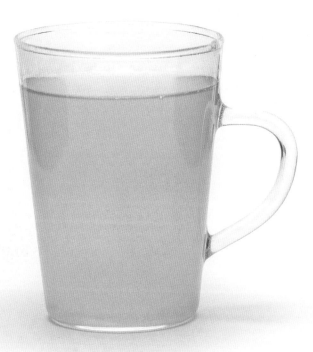

Combine all the ingredients in a teapot with 2¼ cups hot water and steep for 10 minutes. Strain and serve hot. Drink a glass a day until you know your dosage limits.

VANILLA MATCHA LATTE

Serves: 1 - Preparation: 5 minutes

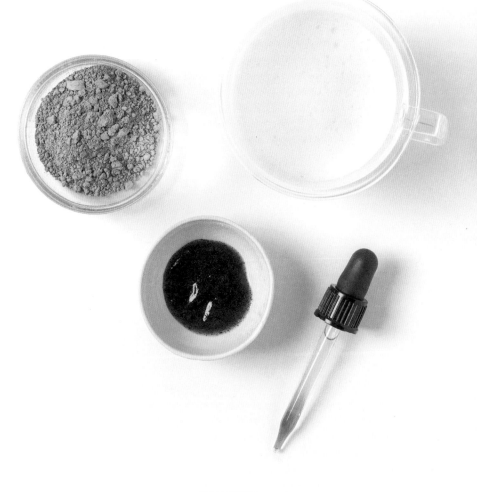

YOU NEED
2¼ teaspoons matcha (green tea) powder • 1 teaspoon vanilla bean paste
22 mg CBD oil (1 dropperful) • 3¾ ounces milk, warmed and frothed

Matcha (green tea) powder contains EGCg, which provides potent cancer-fighting properties.

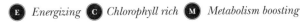 **E** *Energizing* **C** *Chlorophyll rich* **M** *Metabolism boosting*

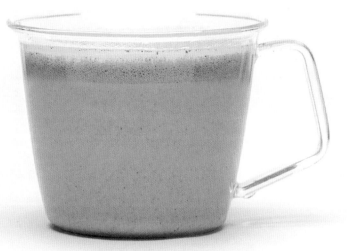

Combine the matcha (green tea) powder with 2 tablespoons hot water and whisk. Add the vanilla bean paste and CBD oil and whisk again. Add the milk and serve hot.

ICED MATCHA WITH MINT

Serves: 1 - Preparation: 5 minutes

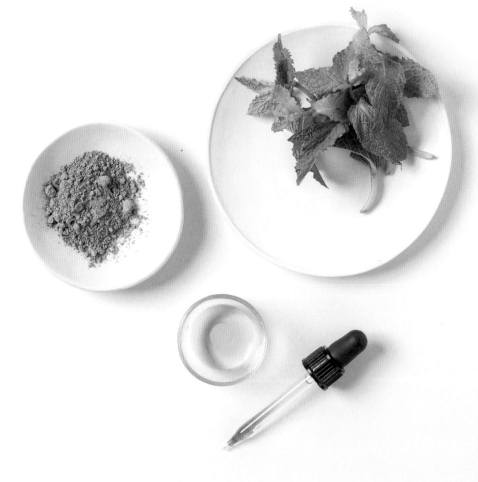

YOU NEED

1½ teaspoons matcha (green tea) powder

3 mint sprigs, leaves picked, plus extra for garnish

1 teaspoon agave syrup • 22 mg CBD oil (1 dropperful)

A refreshing tea packed with antioxidants.

 Detoxifying *Anti-inflammatory* *Concentration boosting*

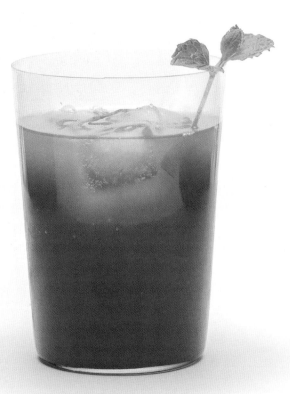

Combine all the ingredients with 1 cup water and ice in a cocktail shaker. Shake until cold, then pour into a tall glass and serve. Garnish with mint.

ICED CITRUS TOASTED BARLEY TEA

Serves: 1 - Preparation: 5 minutes - Steeping: 10 minutes

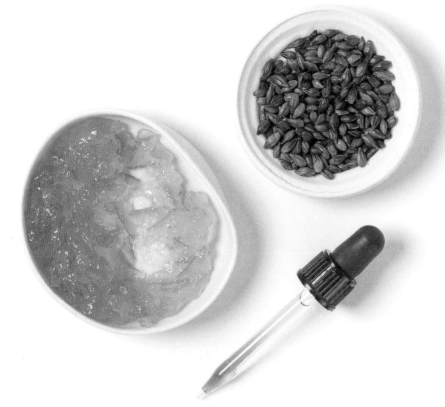

YOU NEED
1 tablespoon toasted barley kernels
2 teaspoons orange marmalade • 22 mg CBD oil (1 dropperful)

This toasty tea can relieve heartburn.

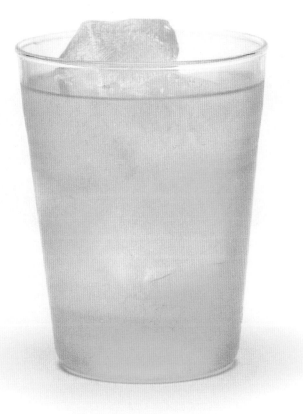

Steep the barley kernels in 1 cup hot water together with the orange marmalade for 10 minutes. Add the CBD oil and stir. Leave to cool to room temperature, then pour over ice. Serve immediately.

LEMON VERBENA & LAVENDER TISANE

Serves: 1 - Preparation: 5 minutes - Steeping: 5 minutes

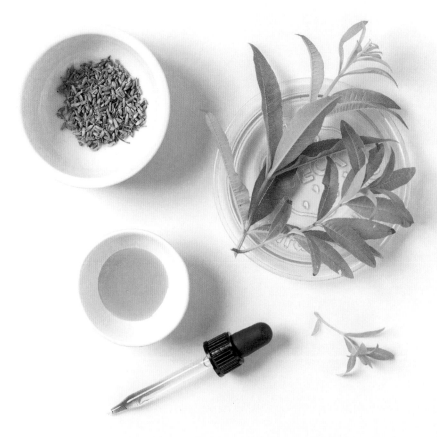

YOU NEED

1 tablespoon dried lemon verbena or 4 fresh sprigs

1 teaspoon dried lavender buds • 22 mg CBD oil (1 dropperful)

½ teaspoon agave syrup or honey, depending on your taste

Lemon verbena can help with digestion.

A *Anxiety relieving*   **T** *Thyroid support*   **S** *Sleep boosting*

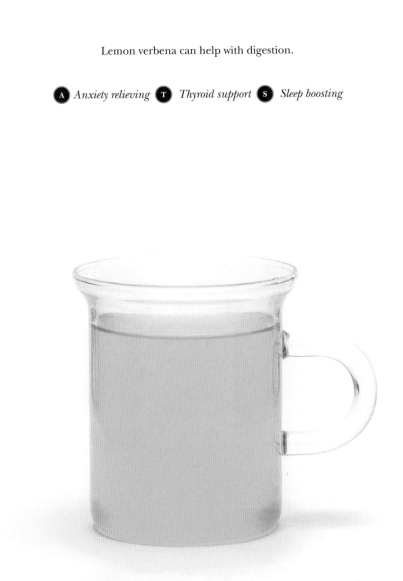

Combine all the ingredients with 8½ ounces hot water and steep for 5 minutes.
Strain and serve immediately.

LICORICE ROOT CHOCOLATE TISANE

Serves: 1 - Preparation: 5 minutes - Steeping: 2 to 3 minutes

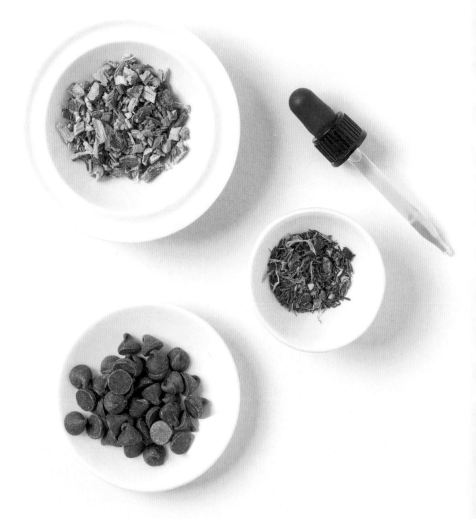

YOU NEED

2 teaspoons dried licorice root • 1 tablespoon chocolate drops
1 teaspoon rooibos tea • 22 mg CBD oil (1 dropperful)

Licorice root can repair the stomach lining and it can relieve food poisoning, heartburn, and ulcers.

 Anti-inflammatory **S** *Stomach calming* **T** *Throat soothing*

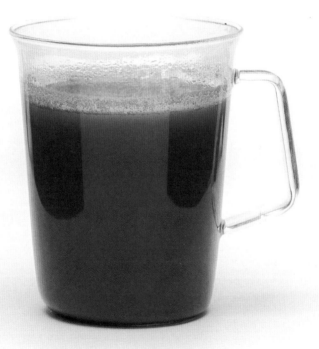

Combine all the ingredients with 8½ ounces hot water and steep for 2 to 3 minutes. Strain and serve immediately.

GOJI, CINNAMON & ANISE TISANE

Serves: 4 - Preparation: 5 minutes - Cooking: 15 minutes

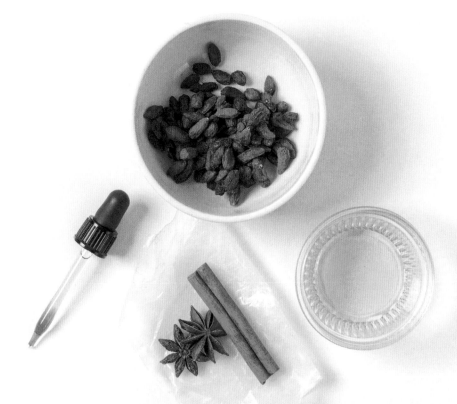

YOU NEED

3 tablespoons dried goji berries • 1 cinnamon stick

2 star anise pods • 1 teaspoon honey

22 mg CBD oil (1 dropperful)

Goji berries may improve energy, mood, and digestive health.

P *Protein rich* **A** *Anti-bloating* **A** *Antidiabetic*

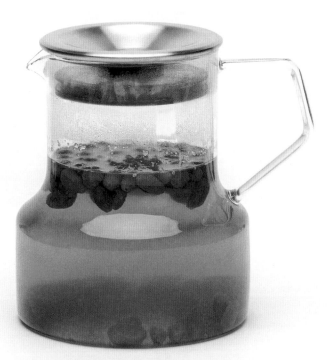

Heat 2½ cups water with the goji berries, cinnamon, and star anise. Simmer for 15 minutes. Pour into a teapot and add the honey and CBD oil. Serve.

FENNEL SEED & APPLE TISANE

Serves: 1 - Preparation: 5 minutes - Steeping: 2 to 3 minutes

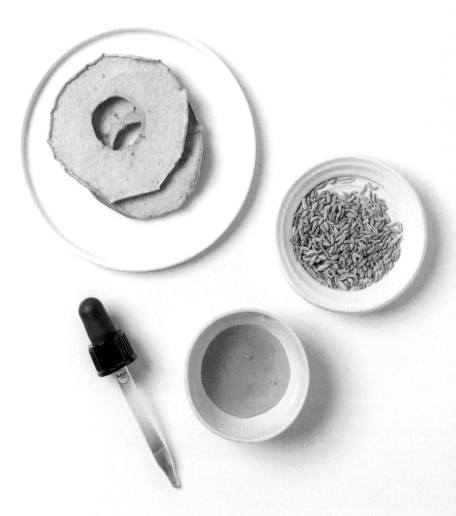

YOU NEED
1 teaspoon fennel seeds • 2 dried apple slices
1 teaspoon honey • 22 mg CBD oil (1 dropperful)

This tea is great for digestion and upset stomachs.

 Antifungal **B** *Blood clot reducing* **R** *Respiratory support*

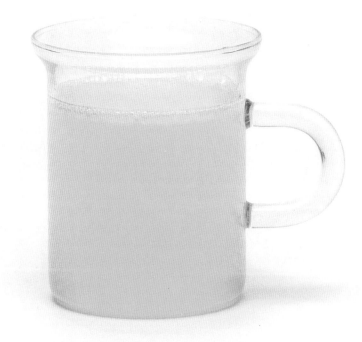

Combine all the ingredients with 8½ ounces hot water and steep for 2 to 3 minutes.
Strain and serve immediately.

ICED VANILLA CHAI LATTE

Serves: 1 - Preparation: 10 minutes - Cooking: 15 to 20 minutes

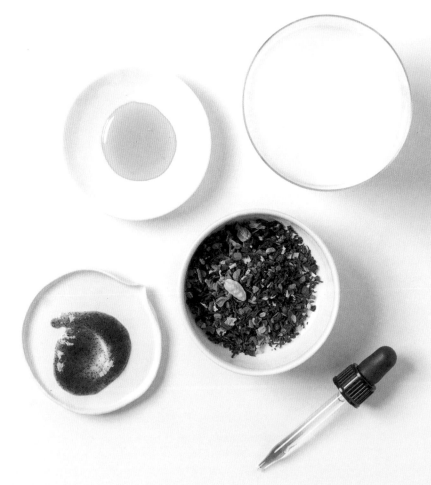

YOU NEED

2 tablespoons chai tea blend • 1 teaspoon vanilla bean paste

1 cup milk or alternative milk • 1 to 2 teaspoons honey

22 mg CBD oil (1 dropperful)

Chai tea boosts heart health and can help reduce blood sugar levels.

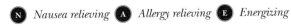 *Nausea relieving* 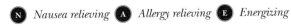 *Allergy relieving* 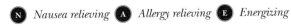 *Energizing*

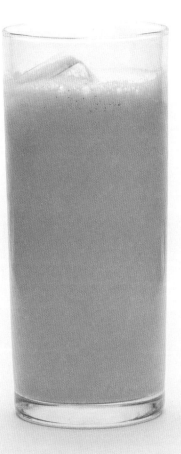

Combine all the ingredients, except for the CBD oil, in a pan and bring to a low simmer. Simmer for 15 to 20 minutes. Strain, add the CBD oil, and stir, then cool. Serve over ice.

ICED MATCHA LEMONADE

Serves: 1 - Preparation: 5 minutes

YOU NEED

1½ teaspoons matcha (green tea) powder • 7 ounces lemonade
22 mg CBD oil (1 dropperful) • 1 lemon wedge

This is packed with antioxidants.

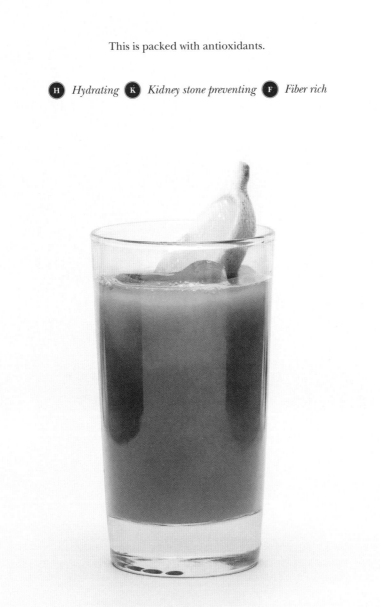

H *Hydrating*   **K** *Kidney stone preventing*   **F** *Fiber rich*

Combine the matcha (green tea) powder and 3½ ounces water in a tall glass and whisk to make a paste. Add ice to fill the glass, then add the lemonade and CBD oil and stir until combined. Serve with the lemon wedge.

IMMUNITY BOOSTER

Serves: 2 - Preparation: 5 minutes

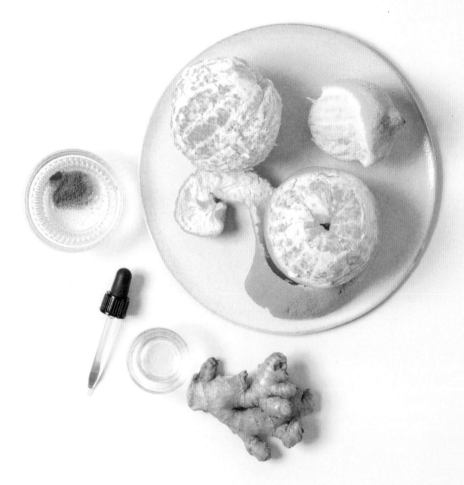

YOU NEED

2 small oranges, peeled • 1 small lemon, peeled

2¼-inch piece of fresh ginger, peeled and chopped • 2 pinches of cayenne pepper

4 drops oregano oil • 40 mg CBD oil (about 2 dropperfuls)

This is great for fighting a cold.

 Antibacterial **R** *Respiratory support* **V** *Vitamin C rich*

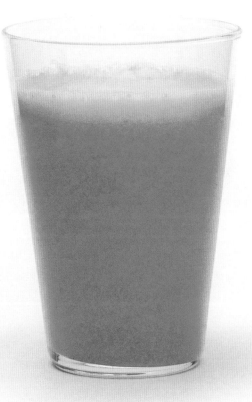

Place the oranges, lemon, and ginger in a juicer and juice. Pour into 2 shot glasses
and divide the remaining ingredients between the glasses. Serve immediately.

DIGESTIVE TONIC

Serves: 2 - Preparation: 5 minutes

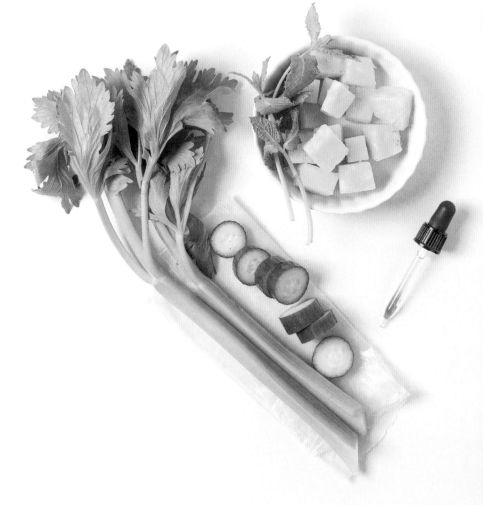

YOU NEED

2 celery sticks • ½ Persian cucumber, chopped
3½ ounces pineapple chunks • 10 mint leaves
40 mg CBD oil (about 2 dropperfuls)

A great alkalizing tonic.

 Anti-inflammatory **M** *Memory boosting* **S** *Skin enhancing*

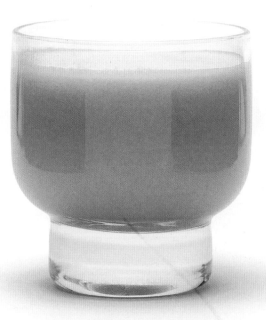

Combine all the ingredients, except for the CBD oil, in a juicer and juice,
then divide between 2 shot glasses. Divide the CBD oil between the glasses and
serve immediately.

CLEANSING TONIC

Serves: 2 - Preparation: 5 minutes

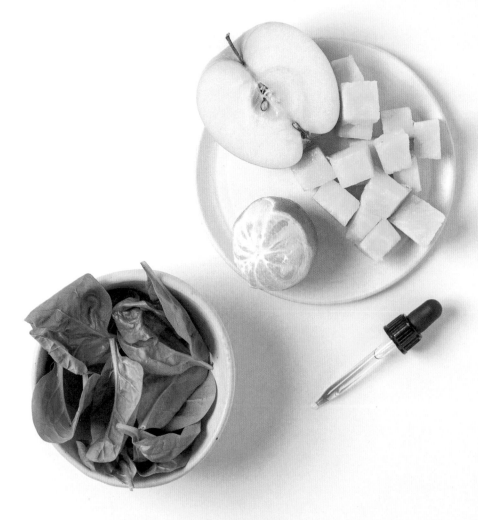

YOU NEED

4 ounces chopped pineapple chunks • 1 ounce spinach

½ Granny Smith apple, chopped

1 lime, peeled • 40 mg CBD oil (about 2 dropperfuls)

A great detoxifying tonic to help purify the body of metals and toxins.

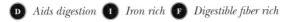 *Aids digestion* **I** *Iron rich* **F** *Digestible fiber rich*

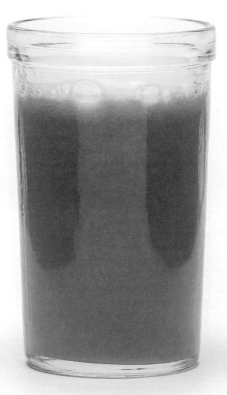

Combine all the ingredients, except for the CBD oil, in a juicer and juice,
then divide between 2 shot glasses. Divide the CBD oil between the glasses and
serve immediately.

INFLAMMATION FIGHTER

Serves: 2 - Preparation: 5 minutes

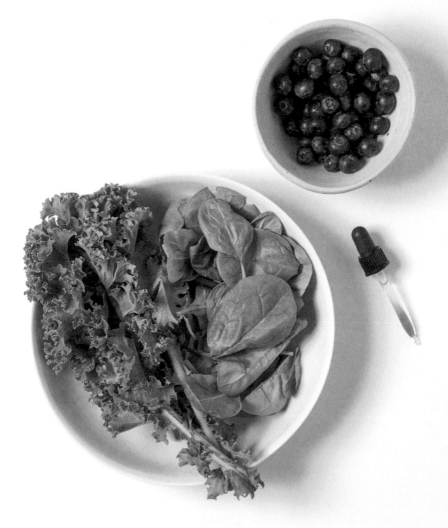

YOU NEED

3 kale leaves, de-stemmed • 1 ouce baby spinach

3½ ounces blueberries • 22 mg CBD oil (1 dropperful)

This tonic is loaded with antioxidants.

 Heart health boosting **B** *Bone strengthening* **B** *Blood sugar stabilizing*

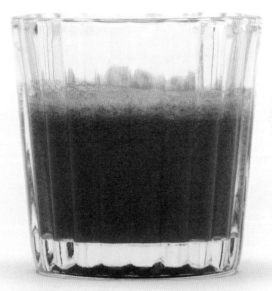

Combine all the ingredients, except for the CBD oil, in a juicer and juice,
then divide between 2 shot glasses. Divide the CBD oil between the glasses and
serve immediately.

HYDRATING TONIC

Serves: 2 - Preparation: 5 minutes

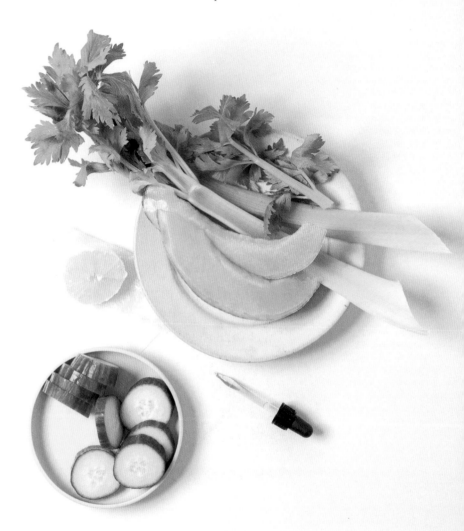

YOU NEED

1 cucumber, chopped • 2 celery sticks

3 ounces cantaloupe, peeled, seeded, and chopped

½ lemon, peeled • 40 mg CBD oil (about 2 dropperfuls)

The cantaloupe in this tonic can boost eye health.

 Beta-carotene rich *Potassium rich* *Bone strengthening*

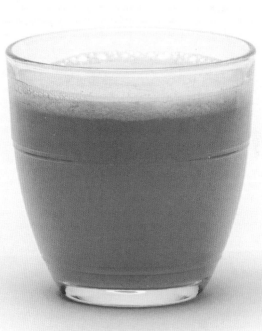

Combine all the ingredients, except for the CBD oil, in a juicer and juice, then divide between 2 shot glasses. Divide the CBD oil between the glasses and serve immediately.

CALMING TONIC

Serves: 1 - Preparation: 5 minutes - Cooking: 10 minutes

YOU NEED

1¼ cups coconut milk • 2 cinnamon sticks
1 teaspoon ashwagandha powder • 1 teaspoon ground turmeric
22 mg CBD oil (1 dropperful)

The ashwagandha powder in this tonic can reduce cortisol levels.

 Anxiety relieving **H** *Heart health boosting* **M** *Metabolism boosting*

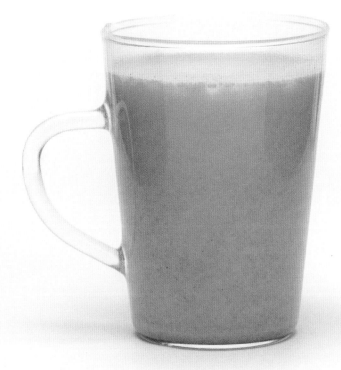

Combine all the ingredients, except for the CBD oil, in a small pan and simmer, whisking occasionally, for 10 minutes. Strain and add the CBD oil. Serve immediately.

SAVORY SNACKS

Adding CBD to your savory snacks will help play with the earthy flavor of the cannabis plant.

Spiced Rosemary Nut Mix • Golden Beet Hummus
Honey Sweet Potato Chips • Cinnamon Spicy Nut Mix
Cheese Ball with Herbs & Nuts • Baked Paprika &
Parmesan Fries • Roasted Red Pepper Dip
Kettle Popcorn • Party Mix

SPICED ROSEMARY NUT MIX

Makes: 215g - Preparation: 15 minutes - Cooking: 20 minutes

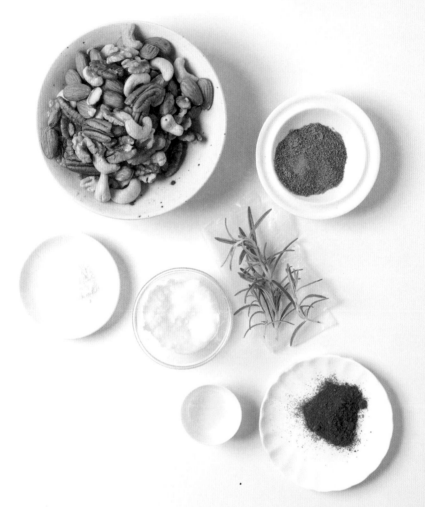

YOU NEED

2 tablespoons coconut oil • 2 tablespoons chopped rosemary

1 tablespoon coconut sugar • 35 mg CBD oil (1½ dropperfuls)

1 teaspoon paprika • 1 teaspoon salt • 7 ounces mixed nuts, such as
cashews, almonds, walnuts, pecans

The nuts in this mix are a great source of healthy fats.

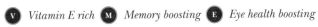 *Vitamin E rich* *Memory boosting* *Eye health boosting*

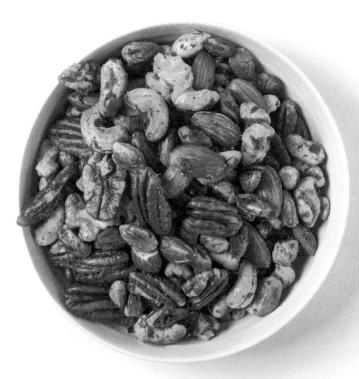

Preheat the oven to 300°F and line a baking sheet with parchment paper. Heat the oil and rosemary in a pan over medium heat for 2 to 3 minutes until fragrant. Add the remaining ingredients, except the nuts, and stir until the sugar is dissolved. In a large bowl, coat the nuts with the rosemary mixture and place on the lined baking sheet. Roast for 15 minutes, then cool completely before serving.

GOLDEN BEET HUMMUS

Serves: 4 - Preparation: 10 to 15 minutes

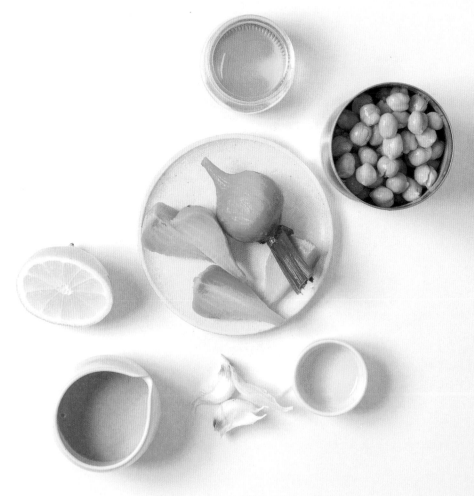

YOU NEED

2 small, roasted golden beets • 2 garlic cloves

15-ounce can chickpeas, drained and rinsed

2 tablespoons tahini • ¼ cup lemon juice • ¼ cup extra-virgin olive oil

35 mg CBD oil (1½ dropperfuls)

Hummus is a great snack item that will help keep you satisfied throughout the day.

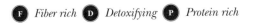 **F** *Fiber rich* **D** *Detoxifying* **P** *Protein rich*

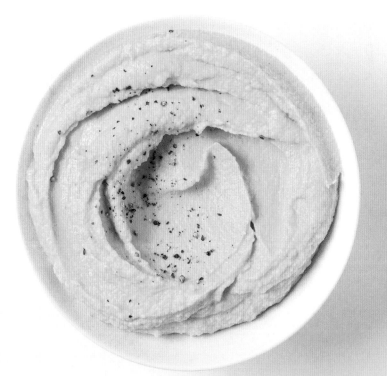

Combine all the ingredients in a food processor and process until smooth, adding water, if necessary. Season to taste.

HONEY SWEET POTATO CHIPS

Serves: 4 - Preparation: 30 minutes - Cooking: 1½ hours

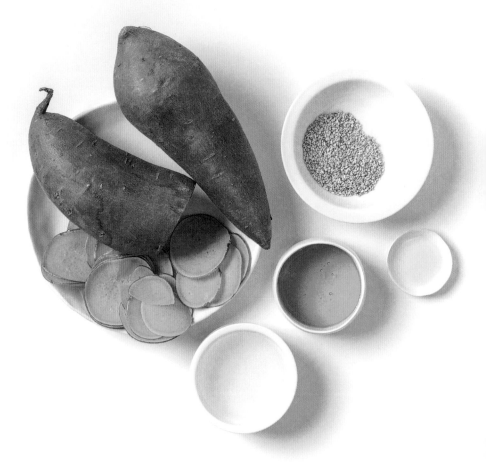

YOU NEED
2 tablespoons coconut oil, melted • 2 tablespoons honey

2 sweet potatoes, thinly sliced on a mandoline (about ⅛ inch)

2 teaspoons toasted sesame seeds • 35 mg CBD oil (1½ dropperfuls)

Sweet potatoes are great for weight loss because of their high fiber content.

 Anti-inflammatory *Vitamin C rich* *Antioxidant rich*

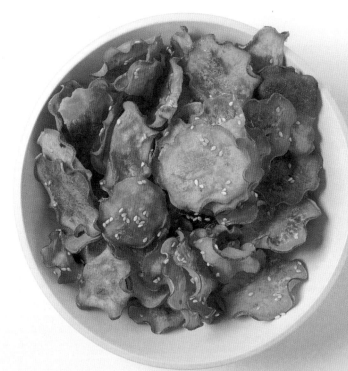

Preheat the oven to 250°F and line a baking sheet with parchment paper. In a large bowl, combine the coconut oil and honey and whisk together until thoroughly combined. Add the sweet potatoes and lightly toss until covered with the honey mixture, then sprinkle with seeds and season with salt. Transfer to the lined baking sheet and bake for 1½ hours, turning and tossing every 30 minutes. Cool completely, then drizzle with the CBD oil and toss to coat.

CINNAMON SPICY NUT MIX

Makes: 215 g - Preparation: 10 minutes - Cooking: 20 to 30 minutes

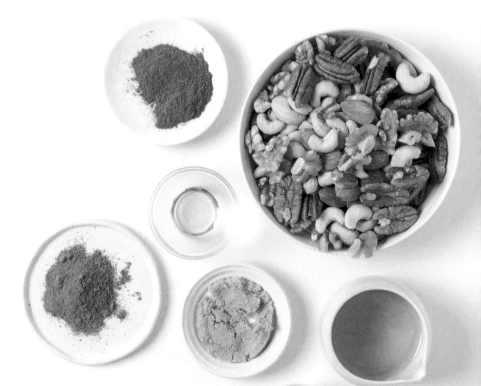

YOU NEED
2 tablespoons olive oil • 1 tablespoon light brown sugar
1½ teaspoons ground cinnamon • 1½ teaspoons cayenne pepper
1 teaspoon salt • 35 mg CBD oil (1½ dropperfuls)
7 ounces mixed nuts, such as cashews, almonds, walnuts, pecans

Nuts are a great snack item because they are low in carbs but high in protein.

 Heart health boosting **P** *Protein rich* **B** *Blood sugar stabilizing*

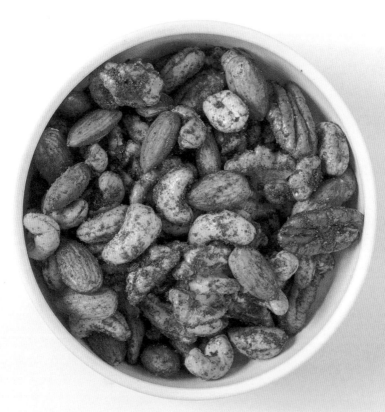

Preheat the oven to 300°F and line a baking sheet with parchment paper.
In a large bowl, combine the olive oil, sugar, seasonings, and CBD oil. Add
the nuts and toss to coat. Roast for 20 to 30 minutes, tossing occasionally.
Cool completely before serving.

CHEESE BALL WITH HERBS & NUTS

Serves: 4 to 6 - Preparation: 1 hour

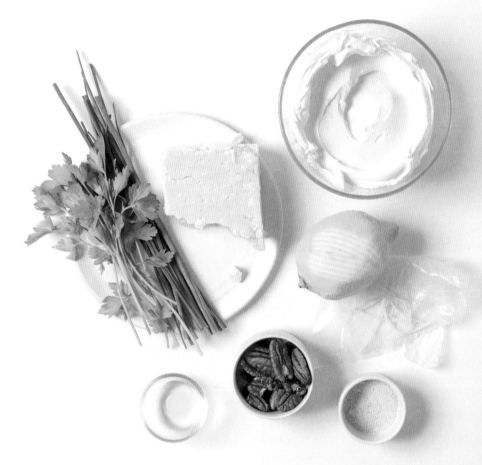

YOU NEED

8 ounces cream cheese, softened • 2¼ ounces finely grated Cheddar cheese

1 teaspoon garlic powder • 60 mg CBD oil (about 3 dropperfuls)

1 teaspoon lemon zest • 3 tablespoons chopped chives

2 tablespoons chopped parsley • 1 tablespoon toasted pecans, chopped

A cheese ball is a great snack with which to get your daily intake of calcium.

 Vitamin D rich P *Protein rich* E *Energizing*

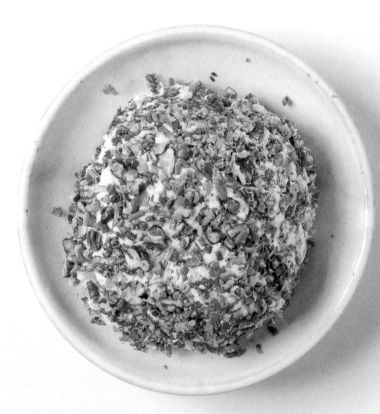

Combine both cheeses, the garlic powder, CBD oil, and lemon zest in a bowl and blend together. Chill for 1 hour, or until firm. Meanwhile, place the herbs and nuts on a plate and toss until combined. Once the cheese is firm, form it into a ball and roll it into the herb and nut mixture. Serve.

BAKED PAPRIKA & PARMESAN FRIES

Serves: 2 - Preparation: 15 minutes - Cooking: 25 to 30 minutes

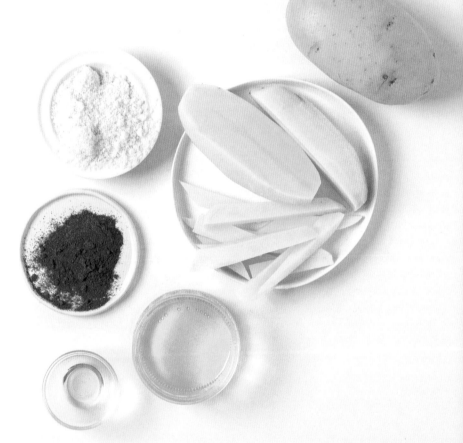

YOU NEED

2 potatoes, such as Yukon gold, peeled and cut into 3⅛ inches long sticks

2 tablespoons olive oil • 2 teaspoons smoked paprika

1 ounce grated Parmesan cheese • 40 mg CBD oil (about 2 dropperfuls)

Potatoes are high in vitamin C, which helps collagen smooth wrinkles.

 Anti-inflammatory **F** *Fat absorbing* **E** *Eye health boosting*

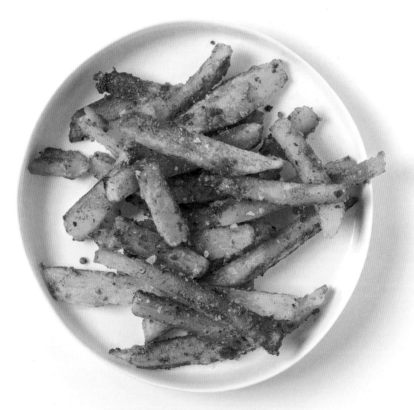

Preheat the oven to 425°F and put a rack in the lower third of the oven. Line a baking sheet with parchment paper. In a large bowl, toss the potatoes with all of the other ingredients, except for the CBD oil, until the potatoes are coated. Place the potatoes in a single layer on the lined baking sheet and bake for 15 to 20 minutes. Remove the baking sheet from the oven and flip the potatoes, and bake for another 10 minutes, or until crispy and cooked. Drizzle the CBD oil on top and toss. Season with salt and serve hot.

ROASTED RED PEPPER DIP

Serves: 2 - Preparation: 15 minutes

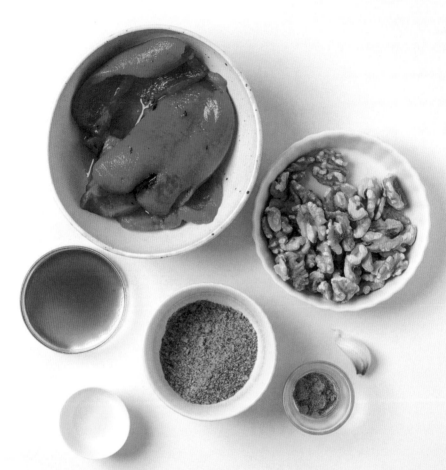

YOU NEED

8-ounce jar roasted red peppers in olive oil, drained

1 garlic clove • 3 tablespoons fresh breadcrumbs

1¾ ounces roasted walnuts • 1 teaspoon pomegranate molasses

½ teaspoon ground cumin • 40 mg CBD oil (about 2 dropperfuls)

Red peppers are great for preventing blood from clotting.

 Vitamin C rich *Omega-3 fatty acid rich* *Diabetes managing*

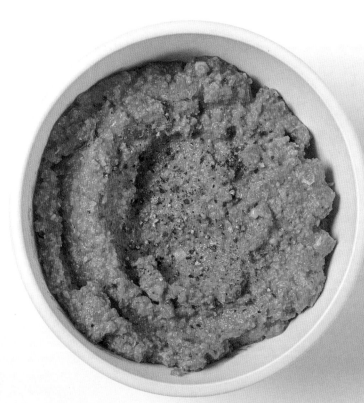

Combine all the ingredients in a food processor and blend until fairly smooth.
Season with salt and serve with pita chips or crudités.

KETTLE POPCORN

Serves: 4 - Preparation: 5 minutes - Cooking: 10 minutes

YOU NEED

2 tablespoons vegetable oil • 2 ounces popcorn kernels

3 tablespoons coconut sugar • ¼ teaspoon salt

35 mg CBD oil (1½ dropperfuls)

A great source of fiber.

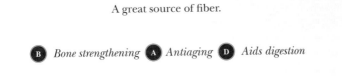

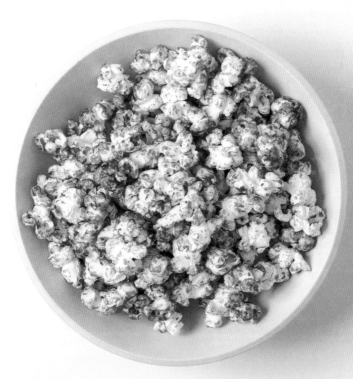

Heat the oil in a large, deep saucepan over medium heat. Once the oil is heated (test with a kernel or two) add the kernels and sugar, then stir and cover with a lid. Once the popcorn starts to pop, keep the pan moving so that the popcorn doesn't burn. Keep shaking pan until the pops start to slow. Place the popcorn in a large bowl and season with the salt. Add the CBD oil and toss to combine.

PARTY MIX

Serves: 4 - Preparation: 10 minutes - Cooking: 30 minutes

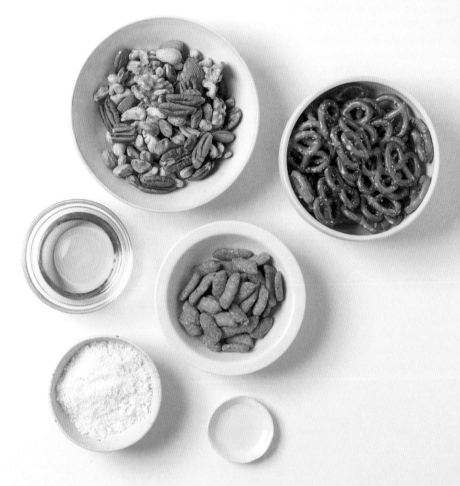

YOU NEED

2¼ ounces pretzels • 4½ ounces mixed nuts, such as pecans, pistachios, cashews

1½ ounces sesame sticks • 1 ounce grated Parmesan

2 tablespoons olive oil • 35 mg CBD oil (1½ dropperfuls)

A great snack that's low in calories.

F *Low in fat* **F** *Fiber rich* **H** *Heart health boosting*

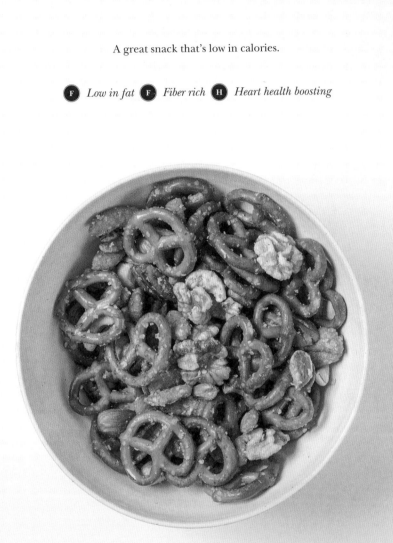

Preheat the oven to 250°F. Line a baking sheet with parchment paper. Combine all the ingredients in a large bowl and toss to coat. Place the mixture on the lined baking sheet and bake for 30 minutes, rotating halfway through. Cool and serve.

SWEET SNACKS

*Date energy balls and chocolates are
some of the recipes found in this chapter,
and they are the perfect vehicles for
CBD oil intake.*

Reishi Nut Chocolate Bark • Chocolate Chip Energy Balls
Caramel Miso Popcorn • Cinnamon Raisin Energy Balls
Ashwagandha Cashew Balls • Strawberry Chia Hand Pies
Vanilla Cashew Frosting • Buckwheat Cake with Frosting
Coconut Cherry Granola Bars • Coconut Cake
Banana "Ice Cream" with Fudge • Coconut & Chocolate
Pudding • Affogato • Banana Bread with Fudge
Fudge & Sprinkles Macaroons • Coconut Maple Cashews

REISHI NUT CHOCOLATE BARK

Serves: 6 to 8 - Preparation: 15 minutes

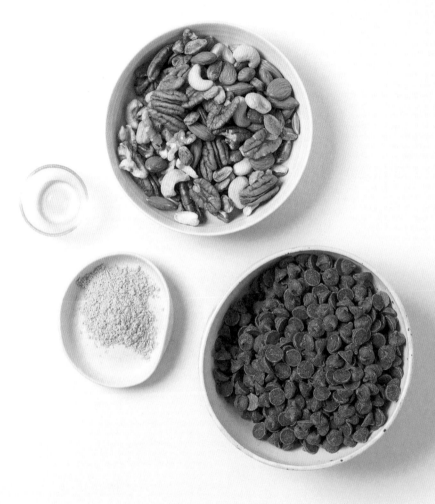

YOU NEED
12 ounces chocolate chips

2 teaspoons reishi powder • 35 mg CBD oil (1½ dropperfuls)

2½ ounces mixed nuts, such as pistachios, pecans, almonds, cashews

Reishi is great for immunity.

 Infection fighting **F** *Fatigue fighting* **V** *Vitamin E rich*

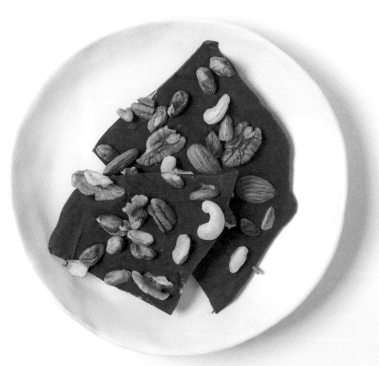

Set a heatproof bowl on top of a saucepan filled with 3½-inch depth of water and bring to a simmer. Add the chocolate to the bowl and melt slowly, about 5 minutes. Once melted, add the reishi and CBD oil and mix thoroughly. Line a baking sheet with parchment paper. Pour the melted chocolate in an even layer on the lined baking sheet. Quickly sprinkle the nuts evenly over the top and cool. Crack the bark into pieces and serve.

CHOCOLATE CHIP ENERGY BALLS

Makes: 6 - Preparation: 15 minutes

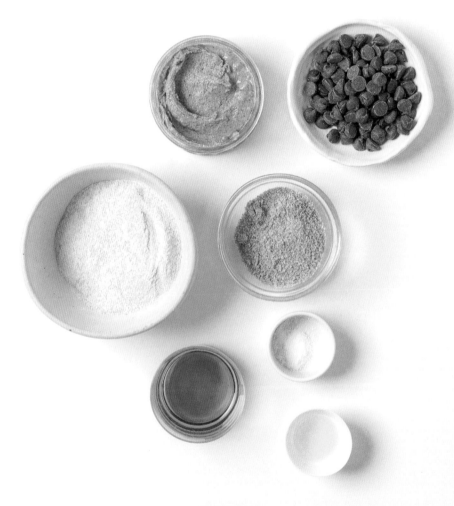

YOU NEED

2¼ ounces almond butter • 3 ounces almond flour

2 tablespoons maple syrup • 2 tablespoons ground flaxseed

45 mg CBD oil (about 2 dropperfuls) • ¼ teaspoon salt • 2¼ ounces chocolate chips

These are rich in omega-3 fatty acids.

B *Blood pressure lowering* **C** *Cancer reducing* **F** *Fiber rich*

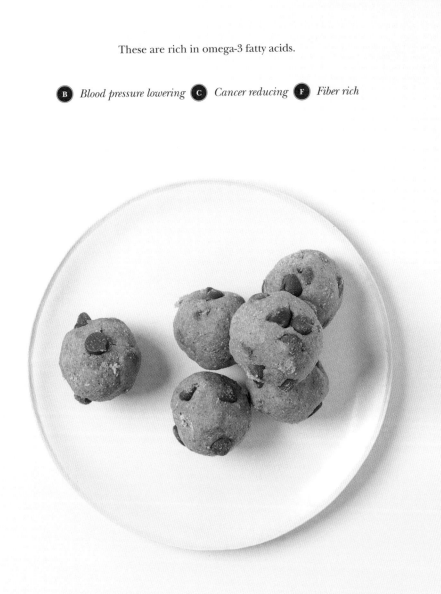

Place the almond butter, flour, maple syrup, ground flaxseed, CBD oil, and salt in a food processor and pulse until combined. Place the mixture in a bowl, add the chocolate chips, and mix together until well distributed. Roll into balls about 2¼ inches in diameter. Store in the fridge or serve immediately.

CARAMEL MISO POPCORN

Serves: 6 - Preparation: 10 minutes - Cooking: 1 hour

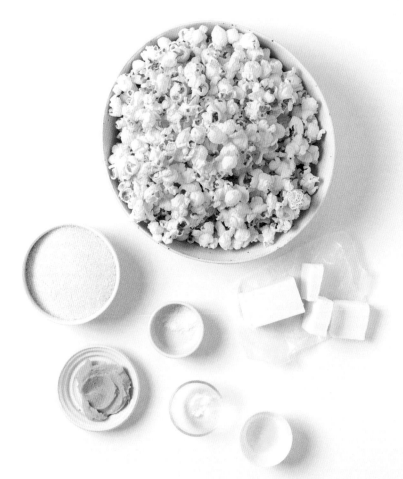

YOU NEED

6 tablespoons unsalted butter • 3½ ounces granulated sugar • ¼ teaspoon salt
1 tablespoon sweet white miso • 35 mg CBD oil (1½ dropperfuls)
pinch of baking soda • 3¼ ounces popped popcorn

Miso is a great probiotic and good for gut health.

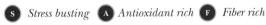 **S** *Stress busting* **A** *Antioxidant rich* **F** *Fiber rich*

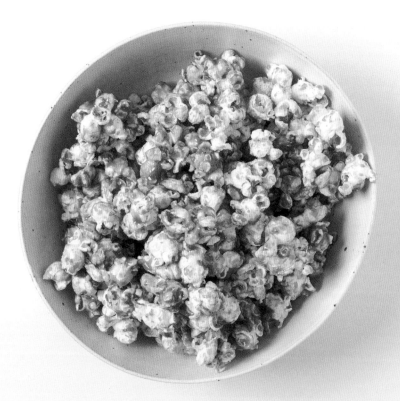

Preheat the oven to 250°F. Line 2 baking sheets with parchment paper. Melt the butter in a pan. Add the sugar and salt and bring to a boil, stirring. Reduce the heat and stir for 1 to 2 minutes until the sugar is dissolved. Remove from the heat and quickly add the remaining ingredients except for the popcorn. Whisk together until well combined. Put the popcorn in a large bowl and pour the caramel over and stir to coat evenly. Place the popcorn in a single layer on the lined baking sheets. Bake for 1 hour, stirring every 15 minutes. Cool completely.

CINNAMON RAISIN ENERGY BALLS

Makes: 6 - Preparation: 30 minutes

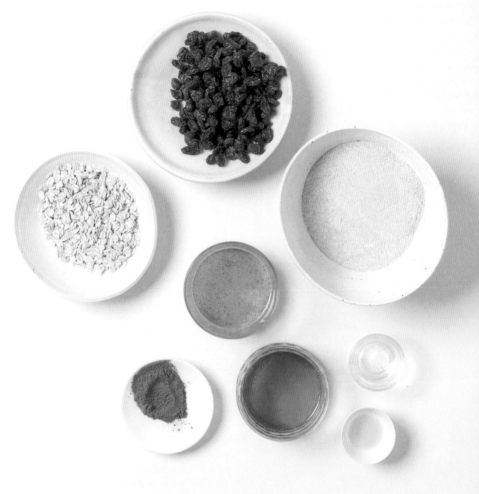

YOU NEED

3 ounces almond flour • 3 tablespoons rolled oats

2¼ ounces almond butter • 3 tablespoons maple syrup

1 teaspoon ground cinnamon • ¼ teaspoon salt

45 mg CBD oil (about 2 dropperfuls) • 1¾ ounces raisins

These can help to boost iron levels.

A *Antiaging* **E** *Energizing* **C** *Cholesterol lowering*

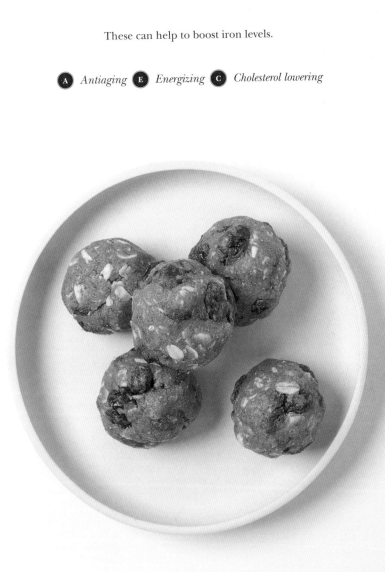

Place all the ingredients except for the raisins in a food processor and pulse until combined. Place the mixture in a bowl, add the raisins, and mix together until well distributed. Roll into balls about 2¼ inches in diameter. Store in the fridge or serve immediately.

ASHWAGANDHA CASHEW BALLS

Makes: 6 - Preparation: 15 minutes

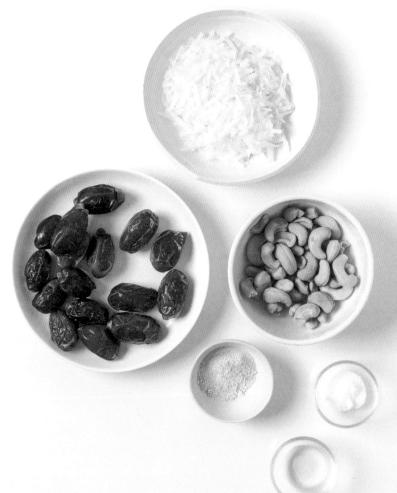

YOU NEED

4 ounces pitted dates • 1¾ ounces raw cashews • 1 ounce desiccated coconut

1 teaspoon ashwagandha powder • ½ teaspoon salt

45 mg CBD oil (about 2 dropperfuls)

Dates are a great source of energy.

 Brain boosting *Blood sugar stabilizing* **S** *Skin enhancing*

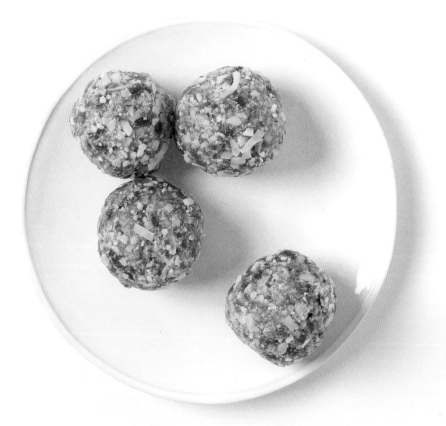

Place all the ingredients in a food processor and pulse until fully combined.
Remove and form into balls about 2¼ inches in diameter. Store in the fridge or
serve immediately.

STRAWBERRY CHIA HAND PIES

Makes: 6 - Preparation: 15 minutes - Cooking: 15 to 20 minutes

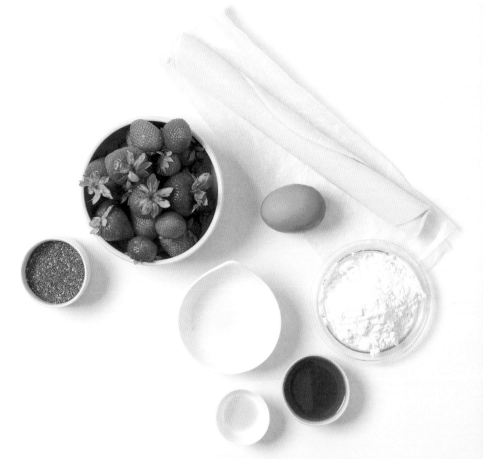

YOU NEED

10½ ounces strawberries, hulled and chopped

2 tablespoons chia seeds • 2 tablespoons maple syrup

1 tablespoon lemon juice • 45 mg CBD oil (about 2 dropperfuls)

1 sheet ready-made shortcrust pastry • handful of all-purpose flour • 1 egg, whisked

These pies are a great source of fiber.

P *Potassium rich* **A** *Allergy relieving* **S** *Skin enhancing*

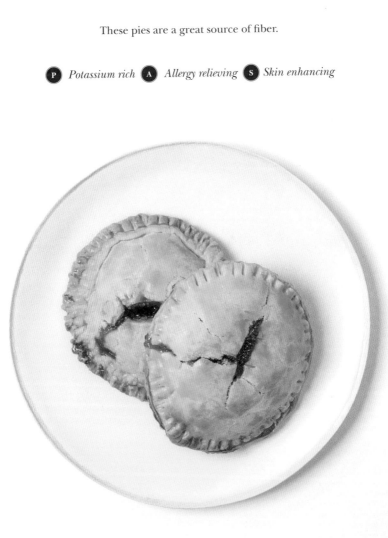

Bring the strawberries, chia seeds, syrup and lemon juice to a low simmer in a pan for 10 minutes. Mash the fruit slightly, remove from the heat, and add the CBD oil. Cool. Preheat the oven to 375°F. Lay the pastry on a floured surface and cut into 4-inch rounds. Chill on a baking sheet. Fill half of the rounds with 1½ teaspoons jam. Brush the pastry edge with some egg, place the remaining pastry rounds on top, and crimp with a fork to seal. Brush with the egg and slit each pie. Bake for 15 to 20 minutes until golden brown. Cool.

VANILLA CASHEW FROSTING

Makes: 3¼ cups - Preparation: 30 to 45 minutes

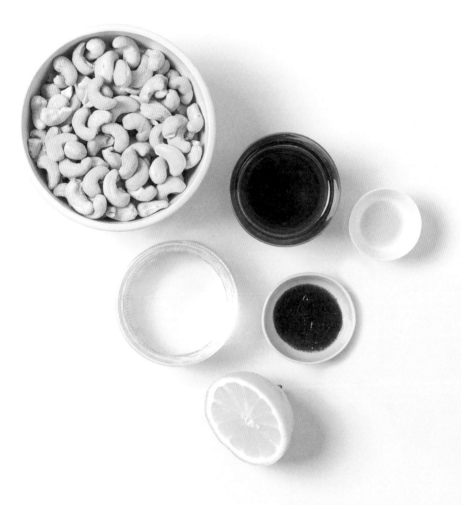

YOU NEED
10½ ounces raw cashews, soaked overnight • ¼ cup coconut oil, melted

3 tablespoons maple syrup • 1 teaspoon lemon juice

1 teaspoon vanilla bean paste • 30 mg CBD oil (about 1½ dropperfuls)

This dairy-free, tangy frosting is a great alternative to buttercream.

 Skin enhancing **I** *Immunity boosting* **B** *Bone strengthening*

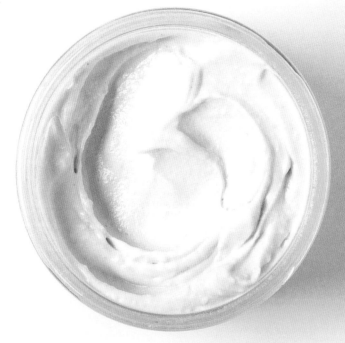

Blend all the ingredients in a high-powered blender until smooth. Chill to firm up.
Frost as needed.

BUCKWHEAT CAKE WITH FROSTING

Serves: 8 - Preparation: 20 minutes - Cooking: 30 to 45 minutes

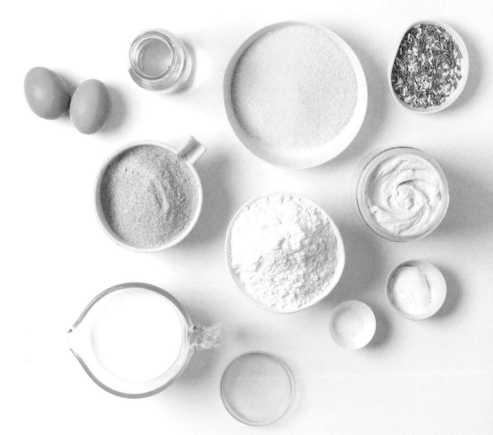

YOU NEED

4¼ ounces all-purpose flour • 6½ ounces buckwheat flour

7 ounces granulated sugar • 1 tablespoon baking powder • ½ teaspoon salt

1 cup whole milk • 6 ounces sunflower oil • 2 eggs, whisked

1 teaspoon vanilla extract • 1 quantity recipe Vanilla Cashew Frosting (page 124)

1 ounce multicolored sprinkles

Buckwheat is high in fiber and protein.

 Magnesium rich **D** *Aids digestion* **I** *Immunity boosting*

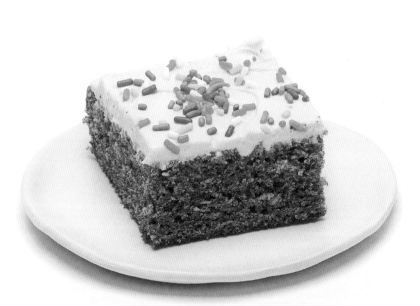

Preheat the oven to 350°F. Grease an 8 x 8-inch baking pan. Sift the dry ingredients
together, except for the sprinkles, into a large bowl. Add the milk, sunflower oil,
eggs, and vanilla and mix until combined; don't overmix. Transfer the batter to
prepared pan and bake for 30 to 45 minutes until a toothpick comes out clean.
Remove from the oven and cool. Frost with the frosting and add the sprinkles on top.

COCONUT CHERRY GRANOLA BARS

Makes: 6 bars - Preparation: 15 minutes - Cooking: 30 to 35 minutes

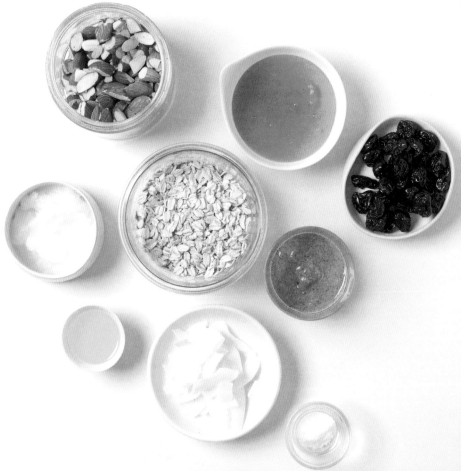

YOU NEED

3¼ ounces rolled oats • 2¾ ounces roasted almonds, roughly chopped

3 tablespoons dried sour cherries • 1 tablespoon unsweetened coconut flakes

½ teaspoon salt • 2 tablespoons coconut oil

30 mg CBD oil (about 1½ dropperfuls) • 2 tablespoons almond butter

¼ cup honey

These are great high-protein, low-sugar bars.

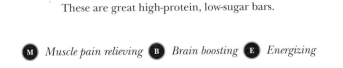

M *Muscle pain relieving* **B** *Brain boosting* **E** *Energizing*

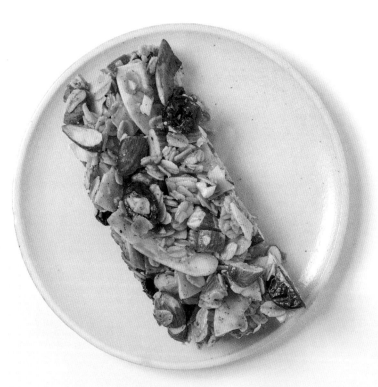

Preheat the oven to 325°F. Line a 13 x 9-inch baking dish with parchment paper. Combine the oats, almonds, cherries, coconut flakes, and salt in a bowl. Heat the coconut oil in a small pan and add the remaining ingredients. Whisk together until combined. Pour over the oat mixture and stir to combine. Pour the oat mixture into the lined baking dish, cover with plastic wrap, press the mixture down, and remove the plastic wrap. Bake for 30 to 35 minutes until golden brown. Cool, then cut into 6 bars.

COCONUT CAKE

Makes: 8-inch square cake - Preparation: 10 minutes - Cooking: 30 to 40 minutes

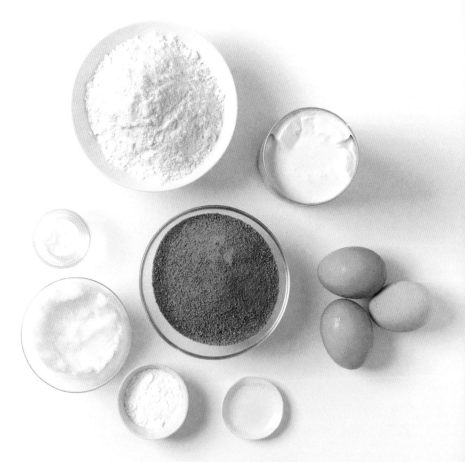

YOU NEED

3½ ounces coconut oil (solid) • 7 ounces coconut sugar • ½ cup canned coconut milk

6¾ ounces all-purpose flour • 3 eggs • 1 tablespoon baking powder

45 mg CBD oil (about 2 dropperfuls) • 1 teaspoon salt

Coconut oil is a great source of energy.

I *Immunity boosting* **E** *Energizing* **M** *Metabolism boosting*

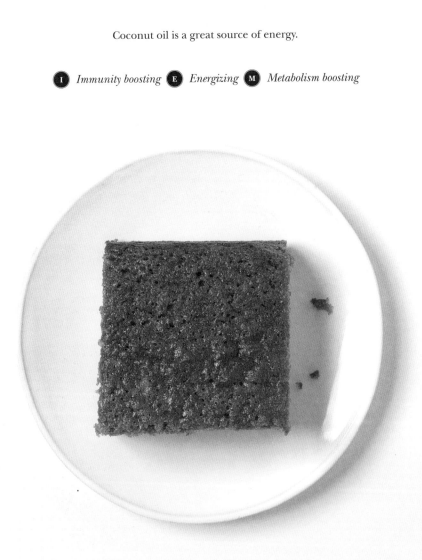

Preheat the oven to 350°F. Grease an 8 x 8-inch baking pan. Beat the coconut oil and sugar together in a large bowl until light and fluffy. Add the remaining ingredients, except for the whipped cream, and whisk together until just combined; do not overmix. Transfer to the prepared pan and bake for 30 to 40 minutes until a toothpick comes out clean. Serve.

BANANA "ICE CREAM" WITH FUDGE

Serves: 2 - Preparation: 45 minutes to 1 hour - Cooking: 10 minutes

YOU NEED
2 ripe bananas, frozen

For the fudge: 2¾ ounces coconut sugar • 4½ teaspoons dark cocoa powder

2 teaspoons unsalted butter • pinch of salt • 1 ounce chocolate chips

2 ounces heavy cream • 30 mg CBD oil (about 1½ dropperfuls)

Cocoa powder can reduce inflammation.

 Anti-inflammatory **P** *Potassium rich* **D** *Aids digestion*

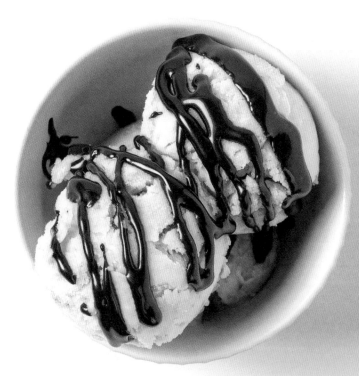

In a food processor, blend the bananas until smooth. Freeze the banana mixture in a container for 1 hour for a firmer "ice cream." Meanwhile, make the fudge. Mix the coconut sugar, cocoa, and a pinch of salt together in a small bowl. Set aside. Heat the butter and chocolate in a saucepan until melted, then add the cream while stirring. Add the dry ingredients and bring to a boil. Remove from the heat, add the CBD oil, and mix to incorporate. Scoop the "ice cream" into 2 bowls and top with the hot fudge.

COCONUT & CHOCOLATE PUDDING

Serves: 4 - Preparation: 15 minutes - Chilling: 3 hours

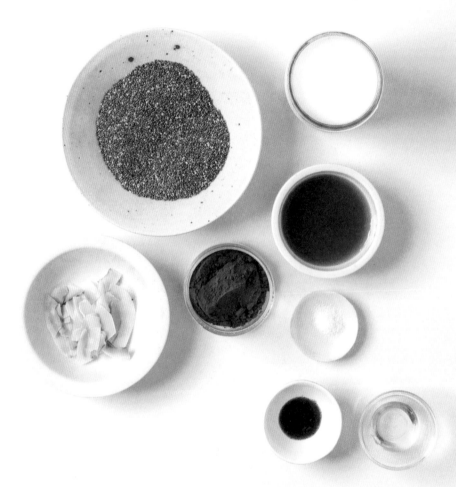

YOU NEED

3 tablespoons cocoa powder • 1 teaspoon vanilla extract

3 tablespoons maple syrup • 8 ounces canned coconut milk

3½ ounces chia seeds • pinch of salt • 80 mg CBD oil (about 4 dropperfuls)

toasted coconut flakes, for topping

Chia seeds are packed with nutrients, including omega-3 fatty acids.

 Antioxidant rich **H** *Heart health boosting* **F** *Fiber rich*

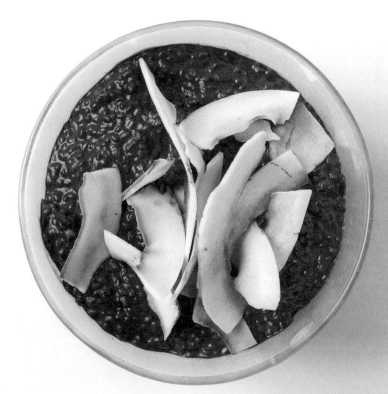

Stir the cocoa, vanilla, and maple syrup together in a bowl until a thick paste forms. Slowly add the coconut milk, a bit at a time, until fully incorporated. Add the chia seeds, salt, and CBD oil and mix. Chill for at least 3 hours. Divide the mixture among 4 cups and top with the coconut flakes.

AFFOGATO

Serves: 1 - Preparation: 15 minutes

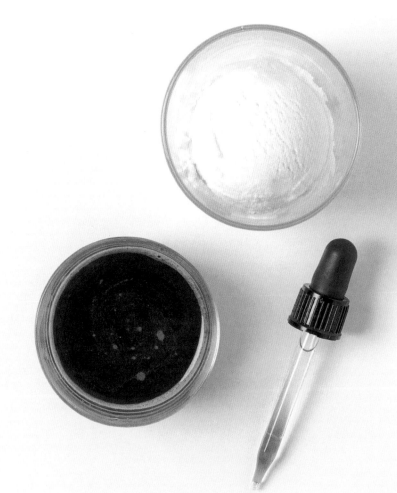

YOU NEED

1 shot espresso • 22 mg CBD oil (1 dropperful)

1 scoop of vanilla ice cream

Espresso has been found to help memory function.

 Immunity boosting **D** *Diabetes risk lowering* **C** *Calcium rich*

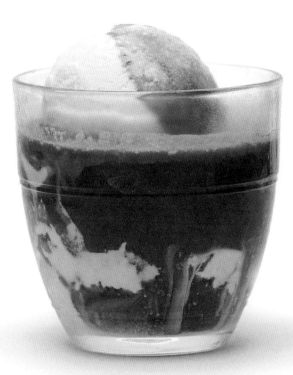

Combine the espresso and CBD oil. Scoop the ice cream into a small glass. Pour the espresso mixture over the ice cream and serve immediately.

BANANA BREAD WITH FUDGE

Makes: 1 loaf - Preparation: 10 minutes - Cooking: 45 to 55 minutes

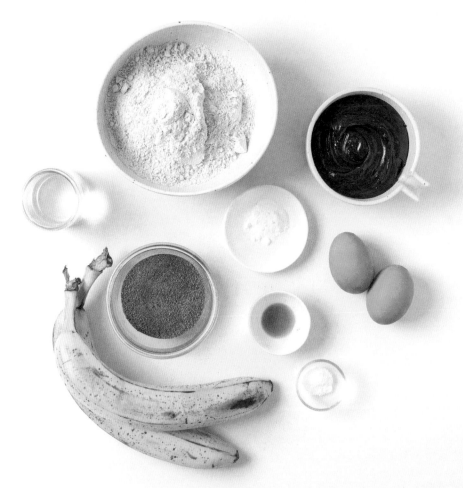

YOU NEED

3 ounces coconut oil, melted, plus extra for greasing • ½ cup coconut sugar

2 eggs, whisked • 2 very ripe bananas, mashed

1 teaspoon baking soda • 1 teaspoon vanilla extract

½ teaspoon salt • 7½ ounces whole-wheat flour

¼ cup Fudge (see page 132)

Bananas can moderate blood sugar levels.

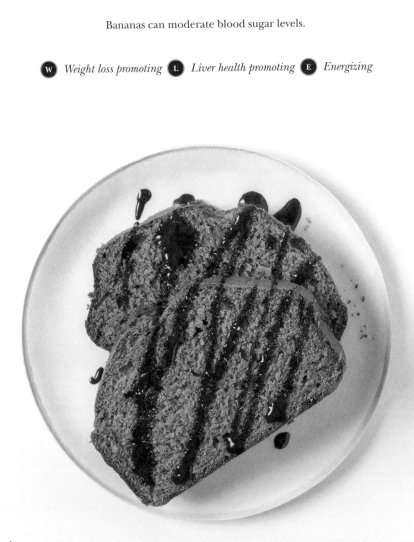

Preheat the oven to 350°F and grease an 8½ x 4½-inch loaf pan. Combine all the ingredients, except for the fudge, in a large bowl and whisk until well combined. Pour into the prepared pan and bake for 45 to 55 minutes until a toothpick comes out clean. Cool. Remove from the pan and drizzle the fudge on top. Slice and serve.

FUDGE & SPRINKLES MACAROONS

Makes: 4 - Preparation: 20 minutes - Cooking: 15 to 20 minutes

YOU NEED

2 large egg whites • ¼ cup granulated sugar

½ teaspoon vanilla extract • ¼ teaspoon salt

4 ounces desiccated coconut • 1 tablespoon honey

3½ ounces Fudge (see page 132) • multicolored sprinkles, for topping

Good-quality honey is rich in antioxidants.

 Weight loss promoting S *Skin enhancing* I *Immunity boosting*

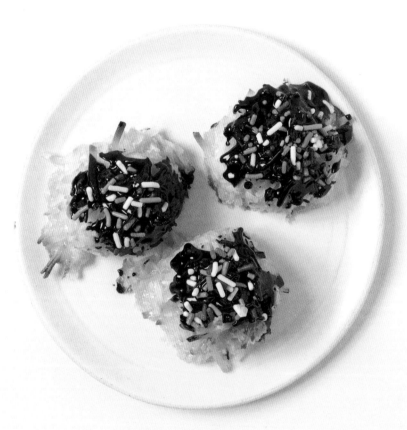

Preheat the oven to 325°F. Line a baking sheet with parchment paper. Combine all the ingredients in a bowl, except for the fudge and sprinkles, and mix until throughly combined. Using an ice cream scoop, scoop the coconut mixture onto the lined baking sheet. Repeat until all of the mixture is used. Bake for 15 to 20 minutes until golden. Cool. Dip in the fudge and sprinkles and place on parchment paper until cool and hardened.

COCONUT MAPLE CASHEWS

Serves: 2 to 4 - Preparation: 10 minutes - Cooking: 5 to 10 minutes

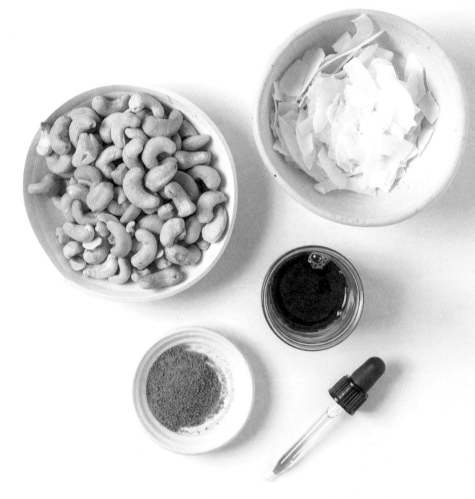

YOU NEED

2¼ ounces unsweetened coconut flakes • 5¼ ounces raw cashews

4 tablespoons maple syrup • 1 teaspoon coconut sugar • pinch of salt

22 mg CBD oil (1 dropperful)

Cashews are great for skin health.

 Heart health boosting **B** *Bone strengthening* **Z** *Zinc rich*

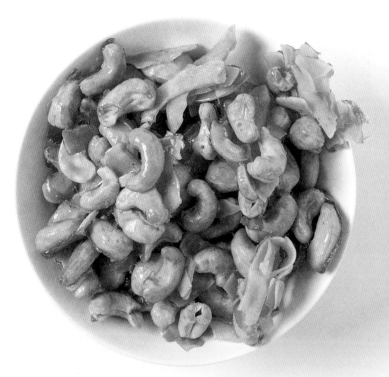

Preheat the oven to 325°F. Line a baking sheet with parchment paper. Mix all the ingredients together with a pinch of salt in a large bowl. Transfer the mixture to the lined baking sheet and spread in a single layer; some clumps are fine. Roast for 5 to 10 minutes until golden brown, stirring halfway through.

HEALTH & BEAUTY

*The recipes in this chapter utilize
CBD oil as a pain reliever and to
reduce inflammation.*

Salve • Lotion

Mood Stabilizer Facial Spray

Scrub • Bath Soak • Healing Cream

SALVE

Makes: 6-ounce container or 3 x 2-ounce containers - Preparation: 15 to 30 minutes
Shelf life: 18 months - Use: Anywhere on the body

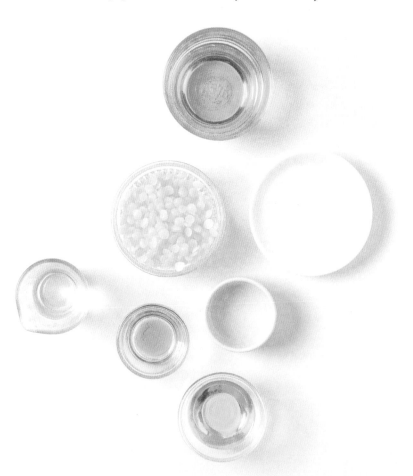

YOU NEED

(300 to 500 mg CBD oil per 1 ounce)

1 ounce beeswax pellets • 1½ ounces arnica oil • 4 teaspoons eucalyptus oil

2 teaspoons vitamin E oil • 2 drops vetiver essential oil

2 tablespoons Leucidal SF Complete

600 mg CBD oil or 3½ teaspoons (based on 1000 mg concentrate)

This salve will aid in soothing muscle soreness and bruises, as well as in healing burns and wounds.

A *Antimicrobial* **A** *Antiviral* **S** *Soothing*

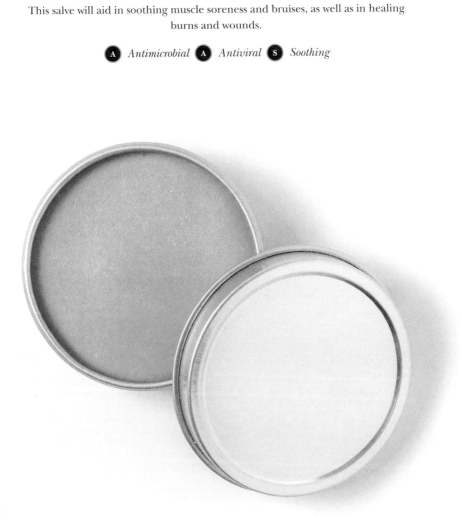

Place the beeswax, arnica, and eucalyptus and vitamin E oils in a double boiler and warm over low heat until the beeswax melts. Remove from the heat, add the remaining ingredients, and stir until well combined. Quickly pour into a 6-ounce container or 3 x 2-ounce containers or a jar and leave to cool completely. Store in a dry, cool place for up to 18 months.

LOTION

Makes: 9 ounces - Preparation: 15 to 30 minutes
Shelf life: 18 months - Use: Anywhere on the body

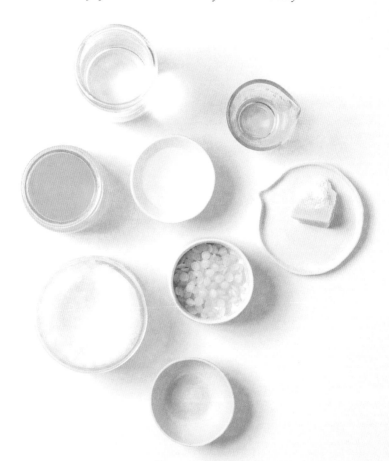

YOU NEED

(300 to 500 mg CBD oil per 1 ounce)

½ cup sunflower oil • ½ cup coconut oil • ¼ ounce cocoa butter

1 tablespoon beeswax pellets • 10 drops calendula oil • ¼ cup distilled water

600 mg CBD oil or 3½ teaspoons (based on 1000 mg concentrate)

2 tablespoons Leucidal SF Complete

CBD oil may help to reduce inflammation.

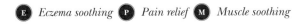 **E** *Eczema soothing* **P** *Pain relief* **M** *Muscle soothing*

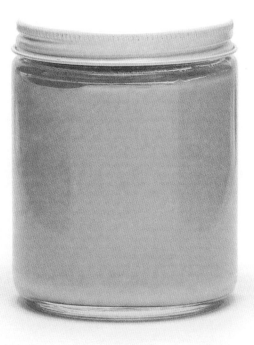

Combine the sunflower oil, coconut oil, cocoa butter, and beeswax in a double boiler and warm over medium heat. Stir until all the ingredients are melted. Remove from the heat and cool to room temperature; it should look creamy. Add the calendula and CBD oils. Using an immersion blender, blend and slowly add distilled water and the Leucidal SF Complete in a steady stream.
Store at room temperature.

MOOD STABILIZER FACIAL SPRAY

Makes: 1 ounce - Preparation: 5 minutes
Shelf life: 1 to 3 months in the fridge - Use: On the face or in the air for aromatherapy

YOU NEED
(300 to 500 mg CBD oil per 1 ounce)
5 teaspoons witch hazel extract • 15 drops bergamot essential oil
15 drops neroli essential oil • 10 drops frankincense essential oil
600 mg CBD oil or 3½ teaspoons (based on 1000 mg concentrate)
4 teaspoons distilled water

This spray can reduce puffiness in the face while reducing stress.

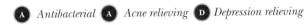 **A** *Antibacterial* **A** *Acne relieving* **D** *Depression relieving*

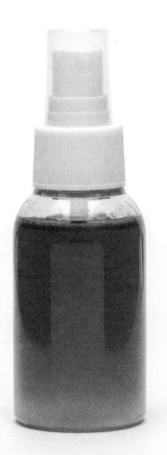

Combine all the ingredients in a small bottle with a mister. Shake the bottle to combine ingredients. Mist on the face to stabilize mood and for a facial refresher. Store in the fridge for up to 3 months.

SCRUB

Makes: 15 ounces - Preparation: 5 minutes
Shelf life: 1 to 3 months in the fridge - Use: Anywhere on the body

YOU NEED
(300 to 500 mg CBD oil per 1 ounce)
15 ounces coarse Himalayan pink salt • 2 tablespoons solid coconut oil
2 tablespoons jojoba oil • 3 tablespoons bentonite clay
3 rosemary sprigs, leaves picked and roughly chopped
5 drops neroli essential oil • 20 mg CBD oil (about 1 dropperful)

CBD oil may help relieve the pain from eczema, arthritis, and psoriasis.

 Anti-inflammatory **P** *Pain relief* **M** *Muscle soothing*

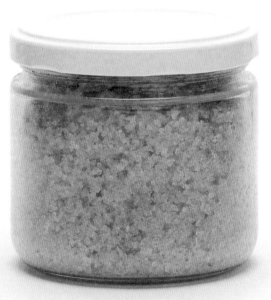

Combine all the ingredients in a jar and mix thoroughly. Use in the bath or shower.
Store in the fridge for up to 3 months.

BATH SOAK

Makes: 9 ounces - Preparation: 5 minutes
Shelf life: 1 to 3 months - Use: Anywhere on the body

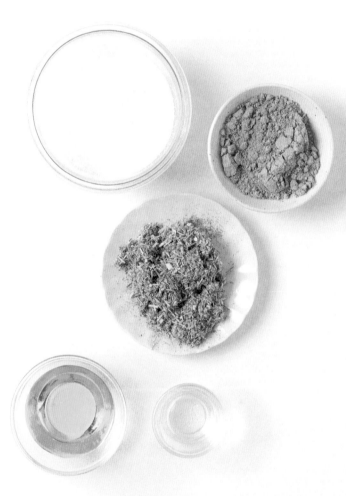

YOU NEED

(300 to 500 mg CBD oil per 1 ounce)

8 ounces Epsom bath salts • 2 tablespoons dried mugwort

1 ounce ginger root powder • 2700 mg CBD oil • 5 drops tea tree essential oil

Mugwort is great for arthritis and joint pain, while CBD oil may help to relieve the pain from eczema, arthritis, and psoriasis.

 Anti-inflammatory **P** *Pain relief* **M** *Muscle soothing*

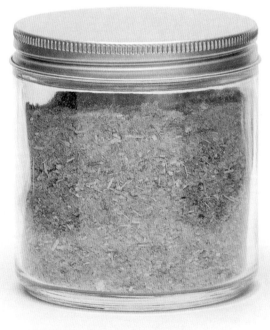

Combine all the ingredients in a jar and mix thoroughly.
Use 2 to 3 tablespoons per bath.

HEALING CREAM

Makes: 11 ounces - Preparation: 15 minutes
Shelf life: 18 months - Use: Anywhere on the body

YOU NEED

(300 to 500mg CBD oil per 1 ounce)

8 ounces cocoa butter • 4 tablespoons jojoba oil

4 tablespoons apricot kernel oil • 3 drops eucalyptus essential oil

1 teaspoon Leucidal SF Complete • 3600 mg CBD oil

CBD oil can help to relieve muscle pain.

A *Anti-inflammatory* **H** *Headache relieving* **P** *Pain relief*

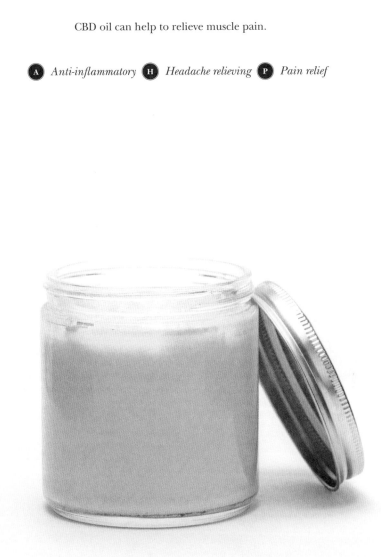

In a double boiler, melt the cocoa butter over low heat. Add jojoba oil and apricot kernel oil and stir to combine. Remove from the heat and add in the remaining ingredients. Transfer to a jar and use for dry skin.

INDEX

Acknowledgements

Thank you to Catie Ziller for asking me to write this book.
Thanks to Kathy Steer for always making sure everything makes
sense and to Tonwen Jones for making it all look good. A
special appreciation to Julia Stotz for sticking through this, and
to my assistant Naomi Bauxprey for making the shoot easy.

The author has researched each plant and superfood used in this book but is not responsible
for any adverse effects any of them may have on an individual. One superfood may be good
for one person but have a negative effect on another. All the superfoods are consumed
entirely at your own risk. Never use anything as an alternative to seeking professional advice.

The information contained in this book is for informational purposes only. It is
not intended as a substitute for the advice and care of your physician, and you
should use proper discretion in utilizing the information presented. The author
and publisher expressly disclaim responsibility for any adverse effects that may
result from the use or application of the information contained in the book.

Published in the United States by Harmony Books, an imprint of Random House,
a division of Penguin Random House LLC, New York.

harmonybooks.com

Harmony Books is a registered trademark, and the Circle colophon
is a trademark of Penguin Random House LLC.

Originally published in French in France by Marabout, a member of Hachette Livre, Paris, in 2020.

Library of Congress Cataloging-in-Publication Data
Names: Hwang, Caroline, author.
Title: The essential CBD cookbook : more than 65 easy recipes for everyday health / Caroline Hwang.
Description: First US edition. | New York : Harmony Books, 2020. | Includes index.
Identifiers: LCCN 2019054976 | ISBN 9780593137543 (paperback) | ISBN 9780593137550 (ebook)
Subjects: LCSH: Cooking (Marijuana) | LCGFT: Cookbooks.
Classification: LCC TX819.M25 H84 2020 | DDC 641.6/379--dc23
LC record available at https://lccn.loc.gov/2019054976

ISBN 978-0-593-13754-3
Ebook ISBN 978-0-593-13755-0

Printed in China

BOOK DESIGN by Tonwen Jones
PHOTOGRAPHY by Julia Stotz
COVER DESIGN by Sonia Persad

10 9 8 7 6 5 4 3 2 1
First US Edition